I0115095

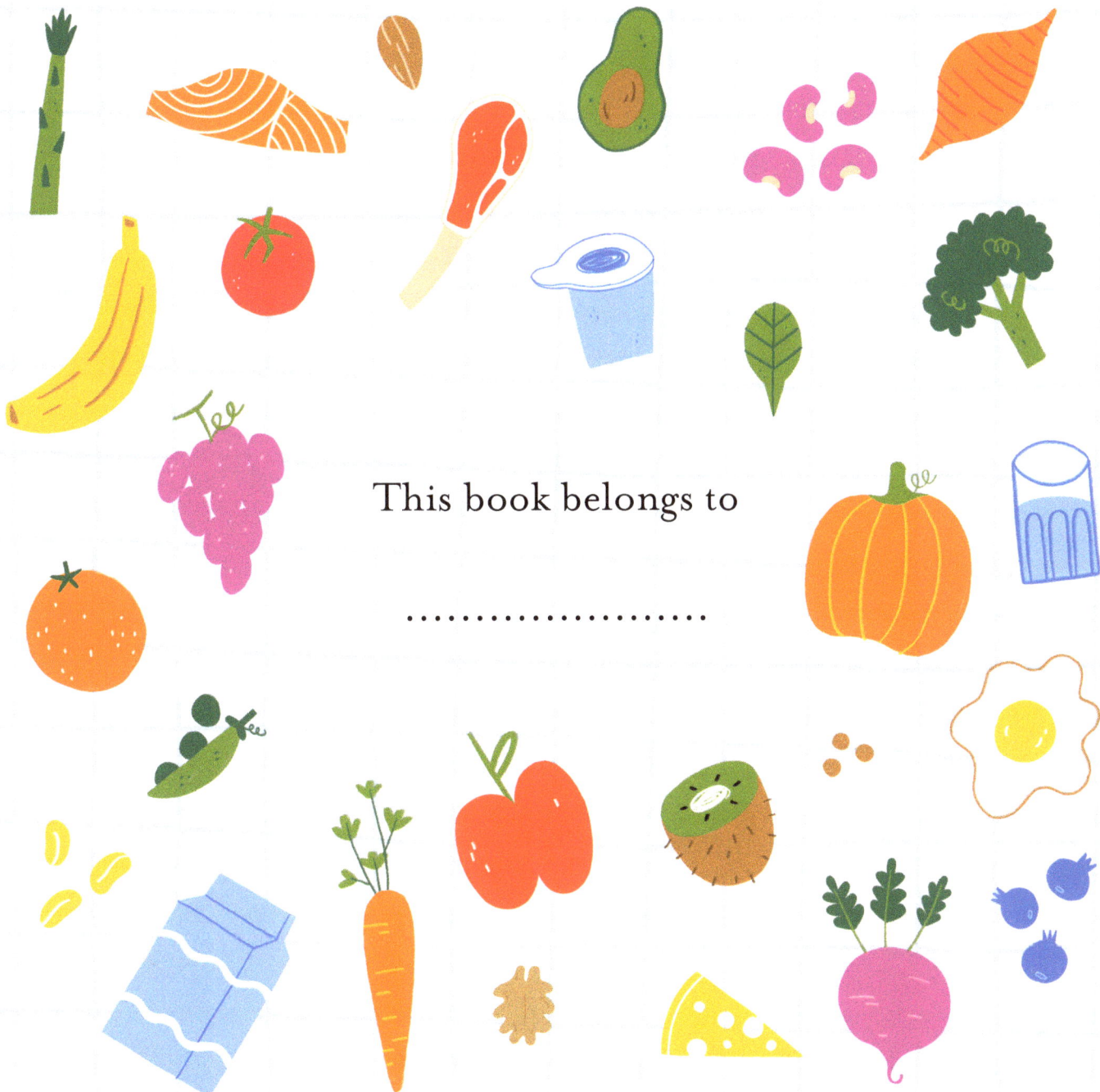

This book belongs to

....

For Heidi, Josie, Leni,
and those still to come.
Our bodies and food
can be so much fun!

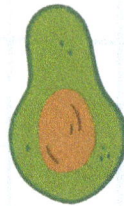

What Does All My Food Do?
Written by Shell Stewart
Illustrated by Claudia Fasser
Copyright © 2024 by Shell Stewart
All rights reserved.
No part of this book may be reproduced in
any manner whatsoever without prior written
permission of the publisher.
First Printing, 2024
Published by Newport Road Press
www.newportroadpress.com.au
ABN 65419524367
ISBN 978-1-7635313-0-7 Hardcover version
ISBN 978-1-7635313-1-4 Paperback version

WHAT DOES ALL MY FOOD DO ?

Written by Shell Stewart

Illustrated by Claudia Fasser

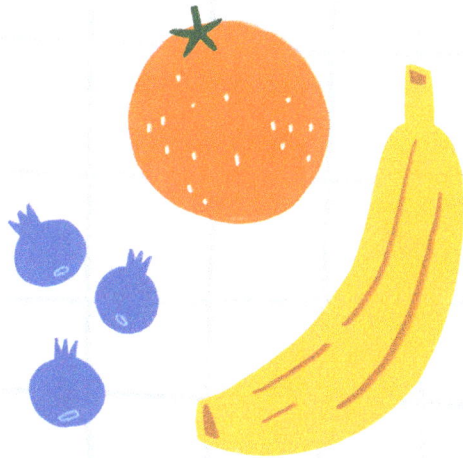

What does all my food do
when I chew and chew and chew?

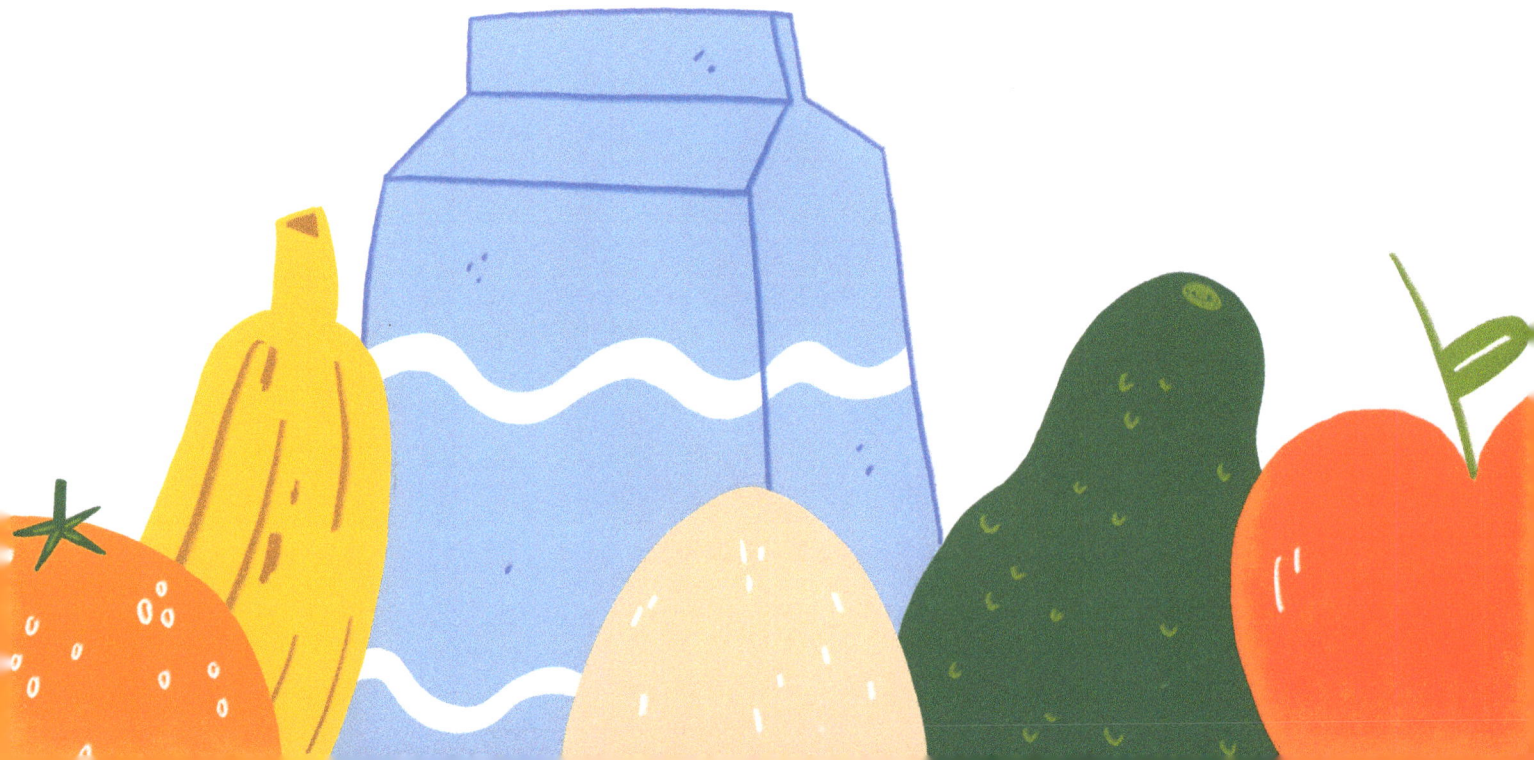

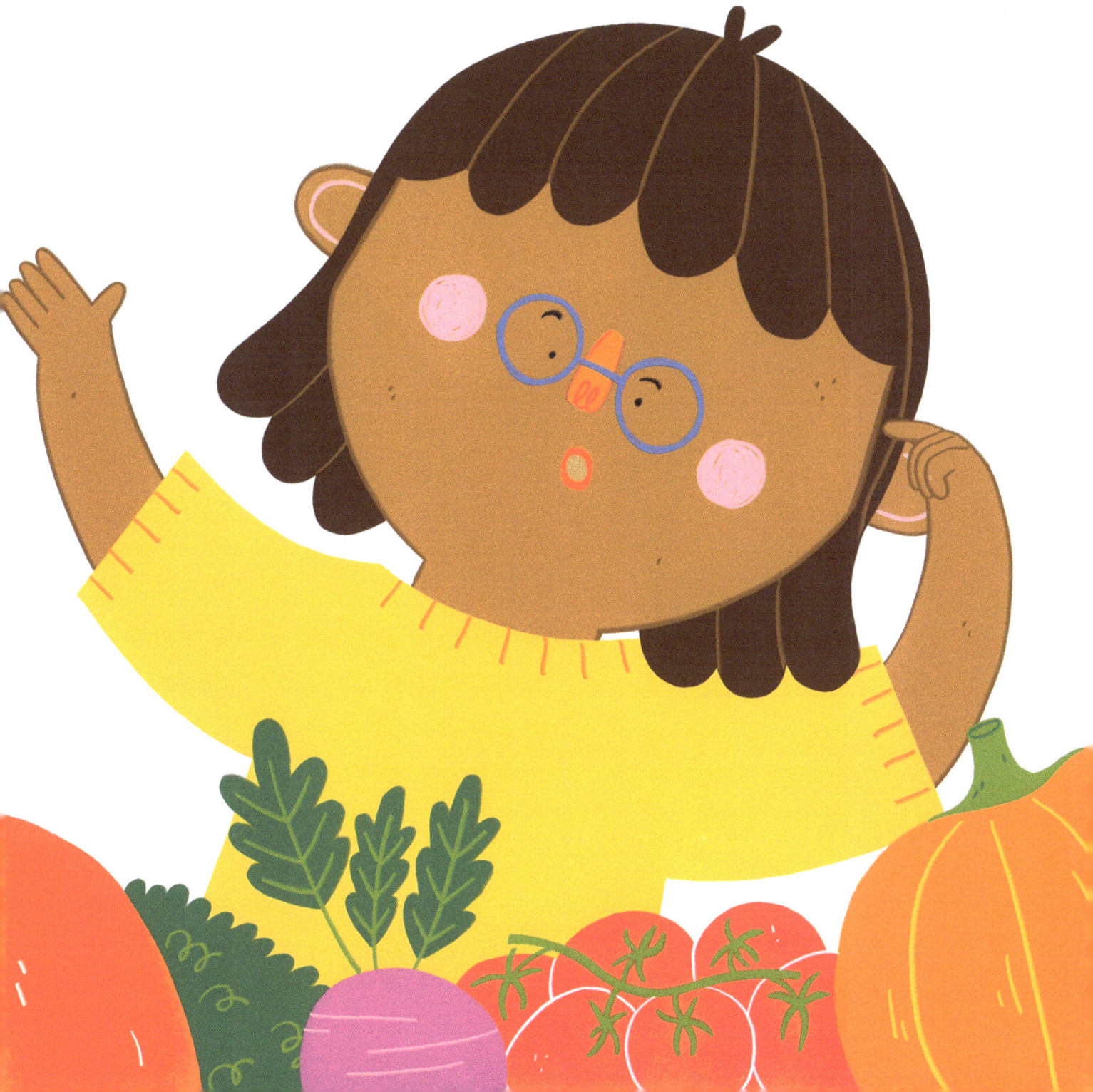

You won't believe it
when I tell you…

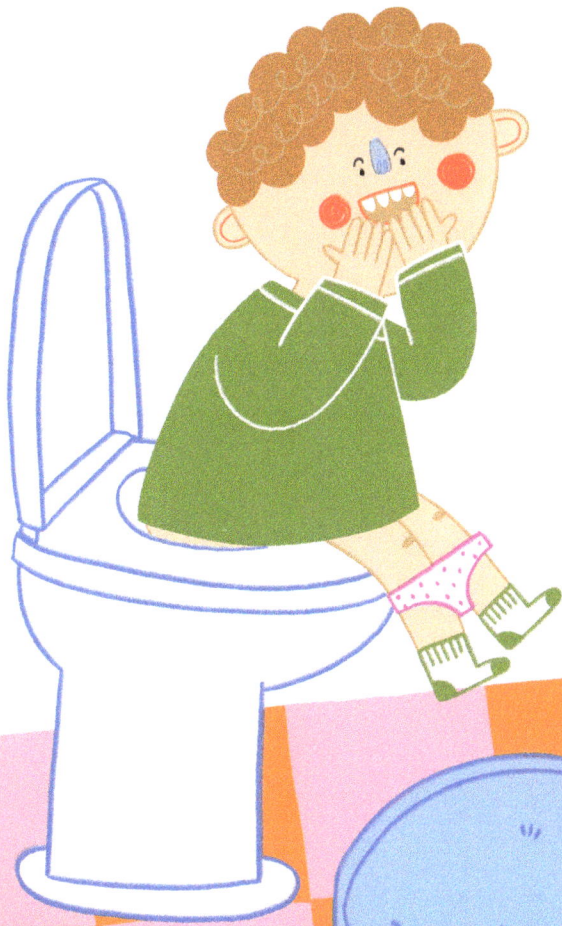

it comes out as... POO.

But before our food turns brown,
it has important jobs to do.

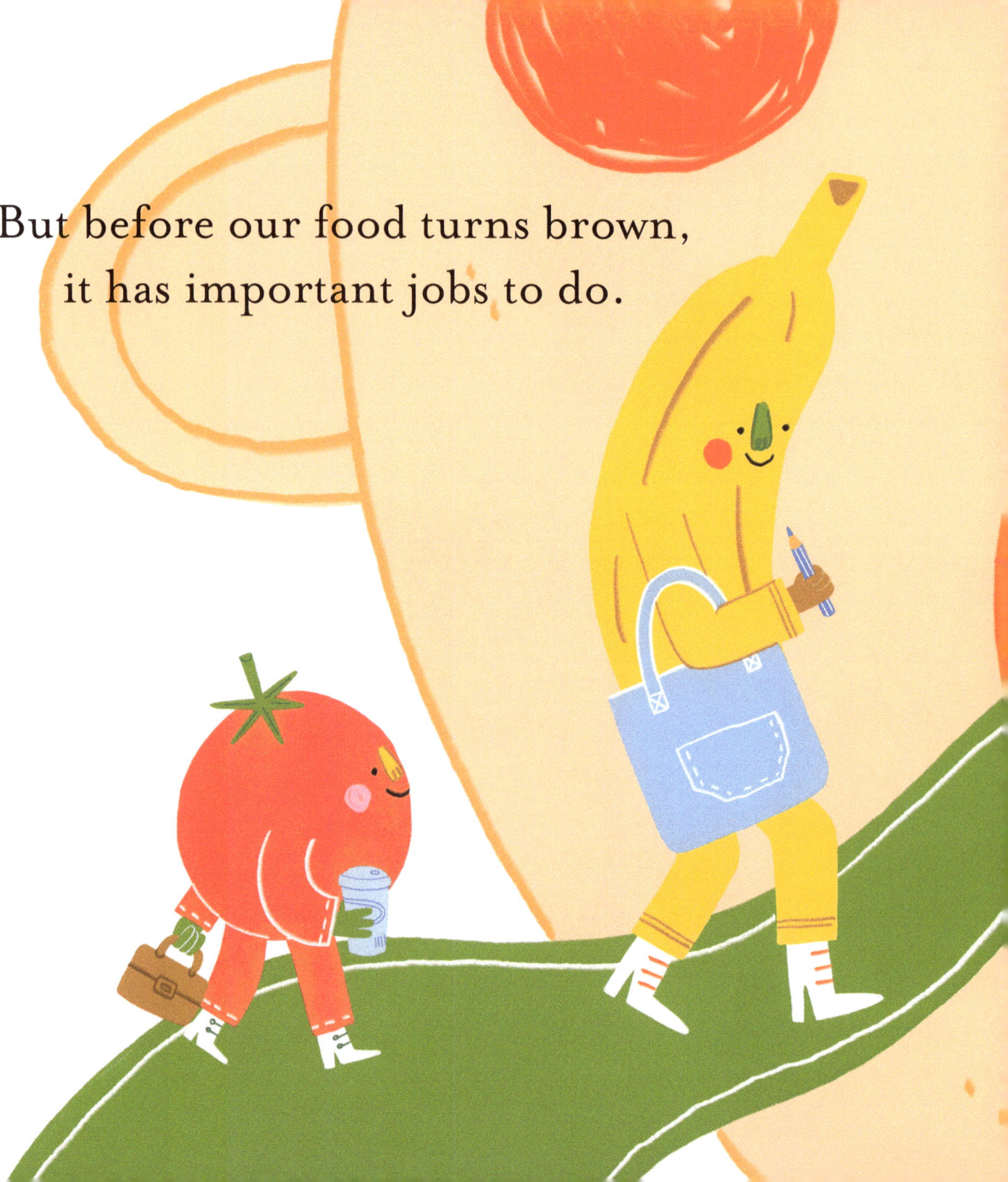

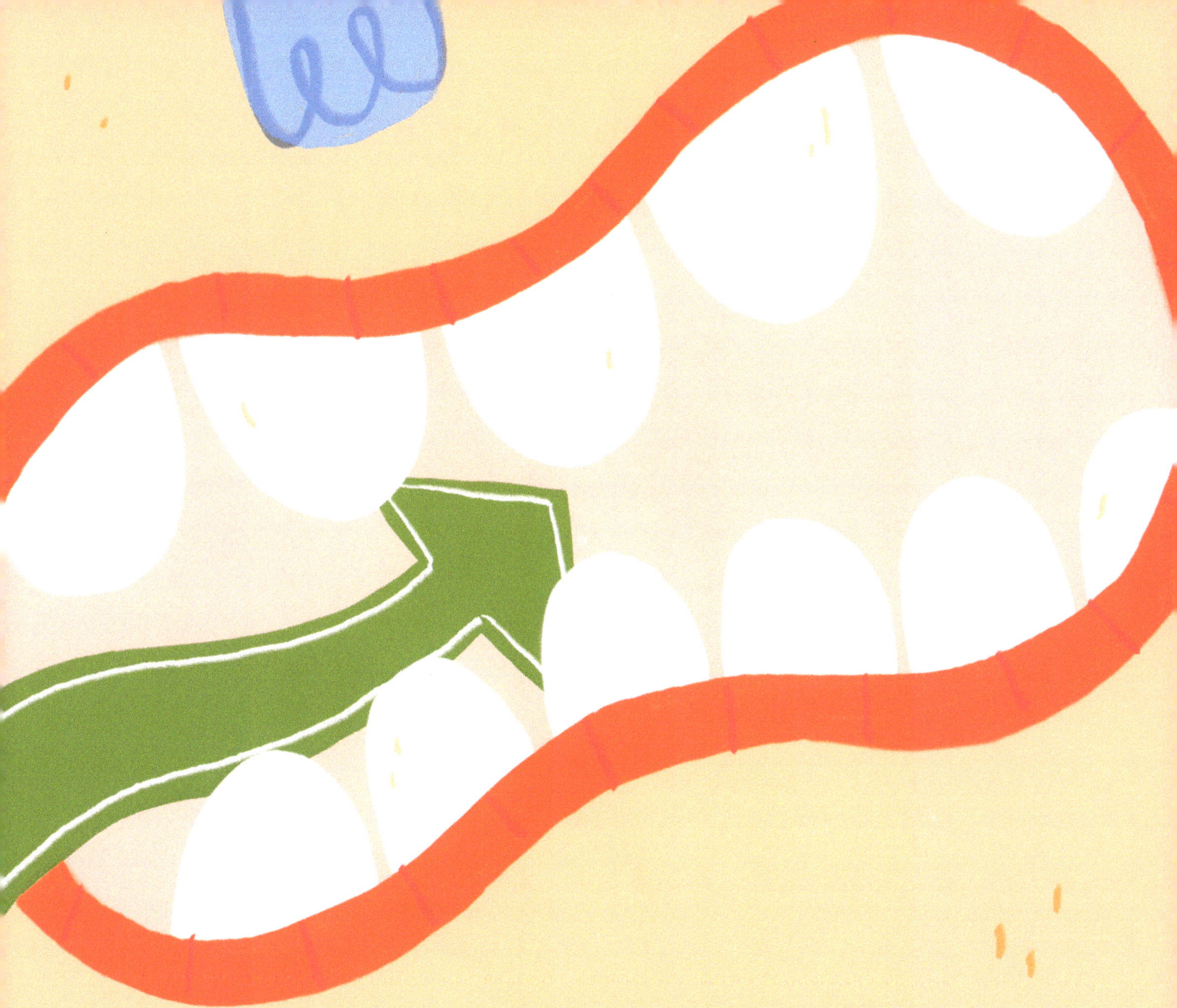

Our yummy food gets straight to work inside me and you!

My oats, salmon and spinach
go down into my tummy.

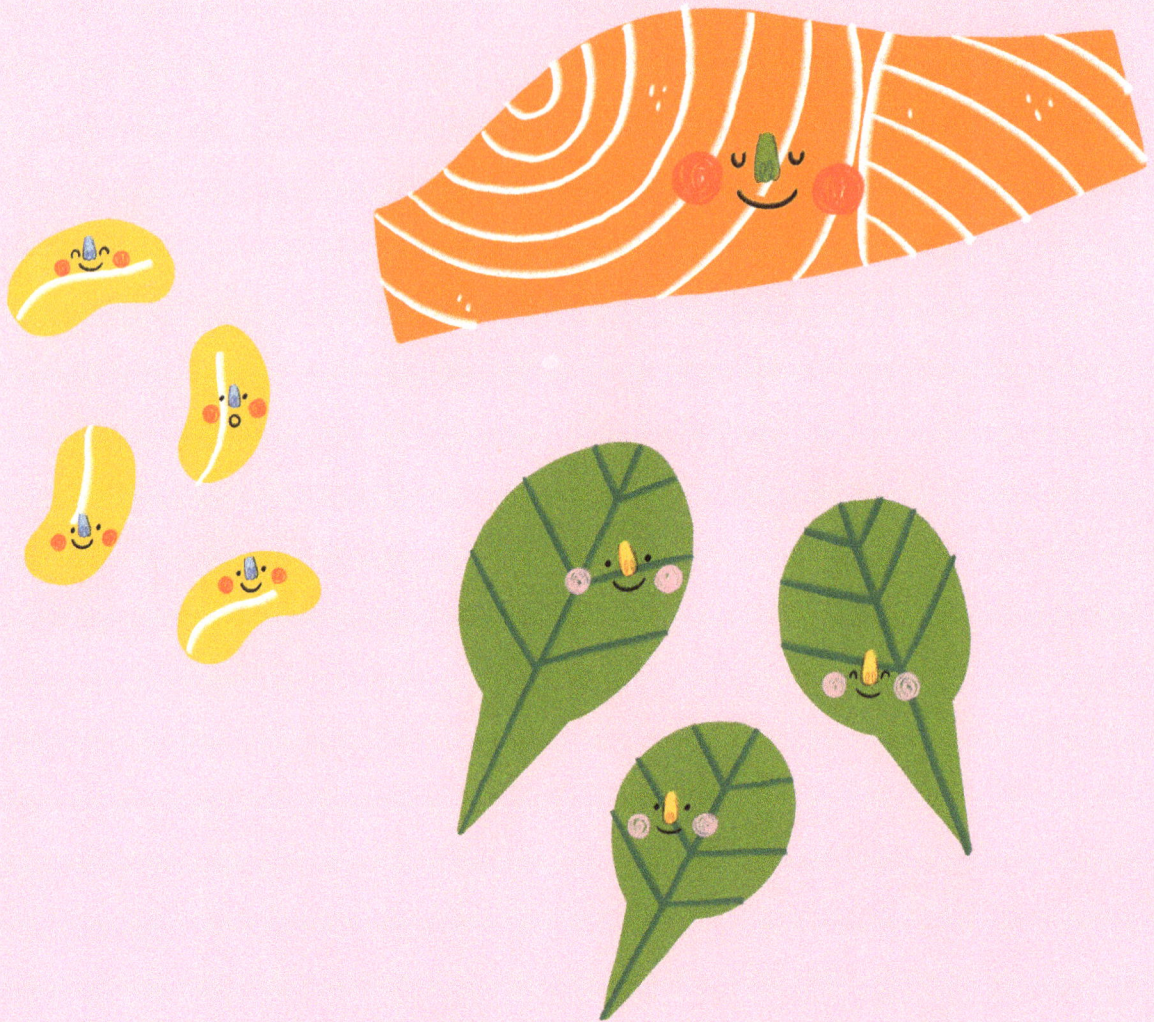

Then what do they do?

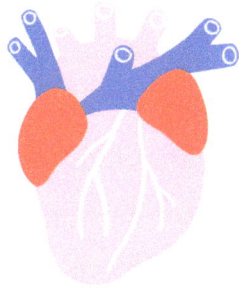

They help my HEART to beat strong
so I can play all day long.

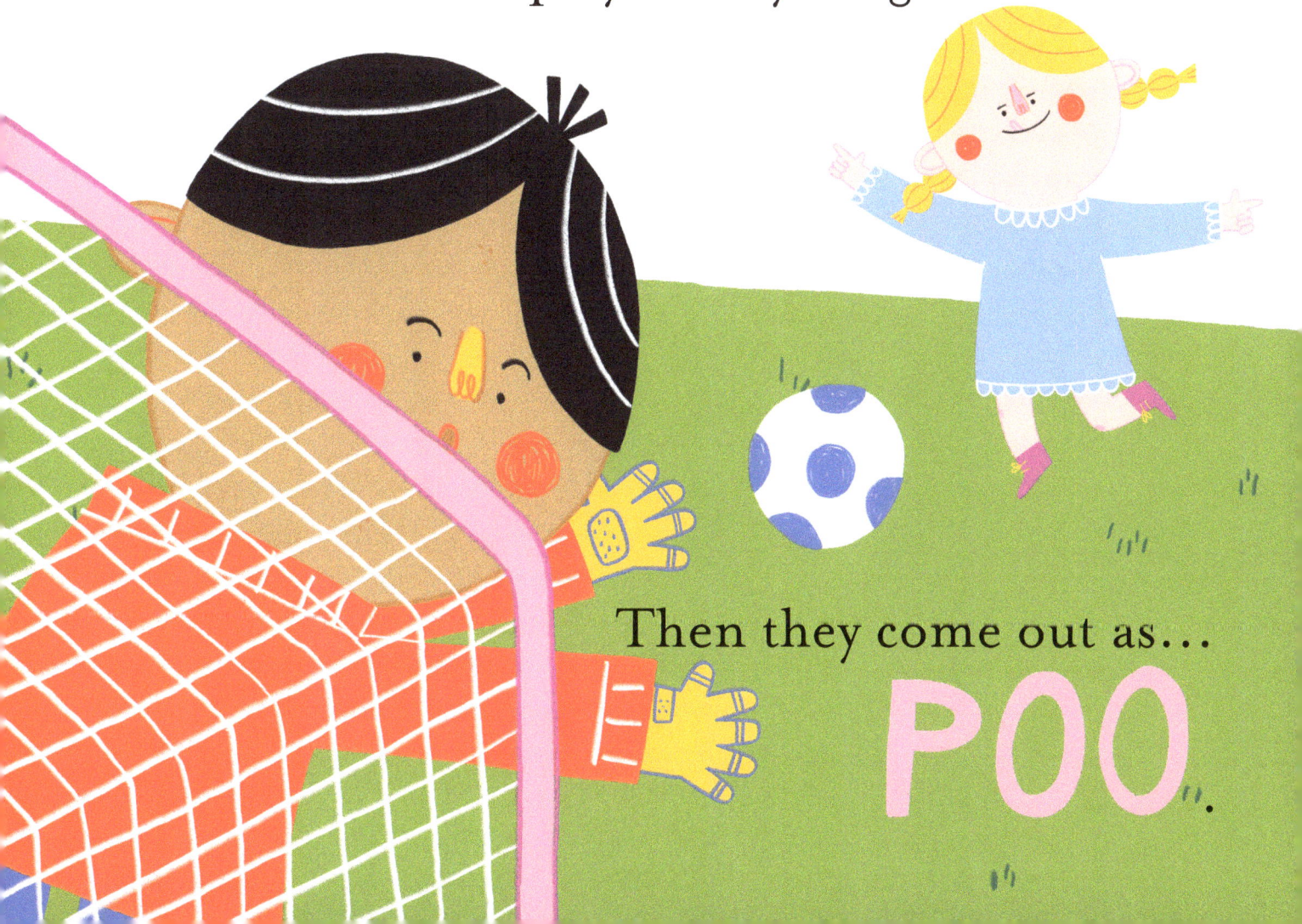

Then they come out as...

POO.

My blueberries, nuts and avocado
go down into my tummy.

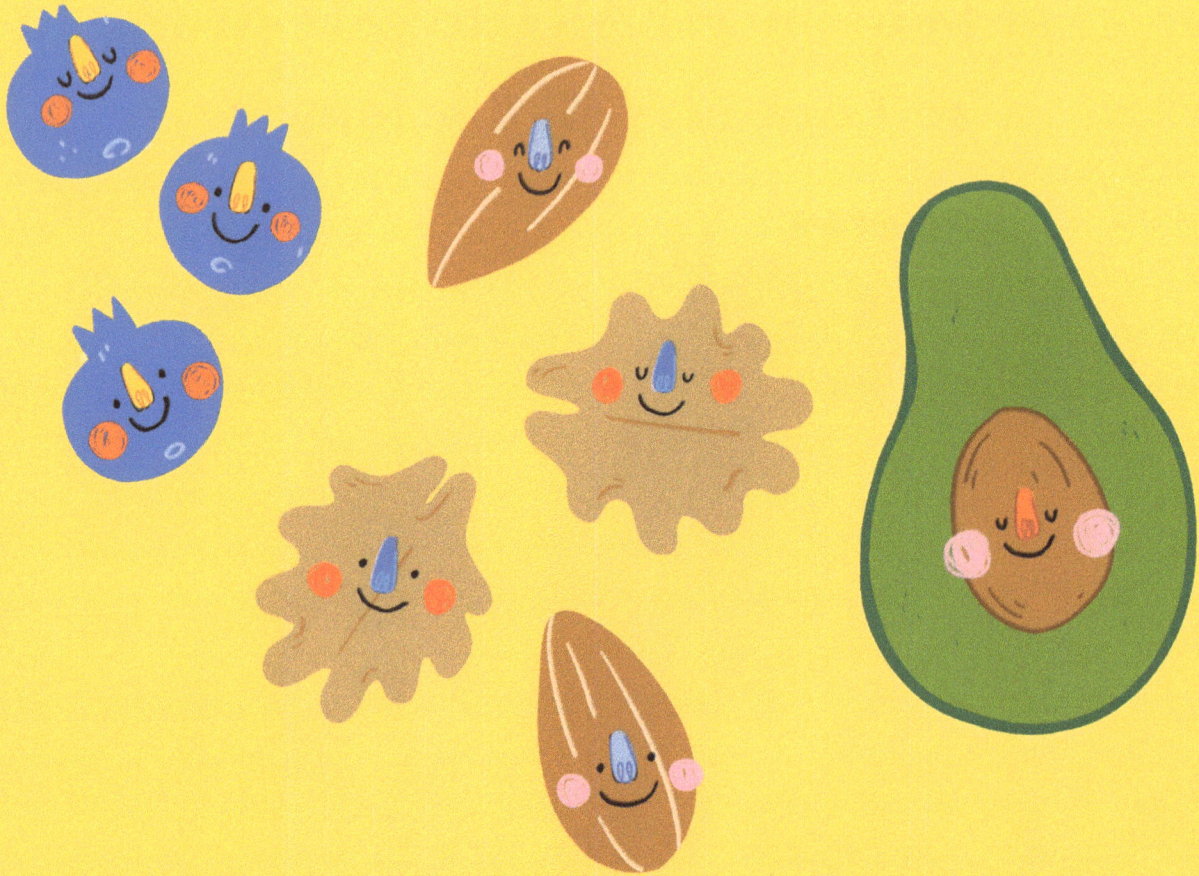

Then what do they do?

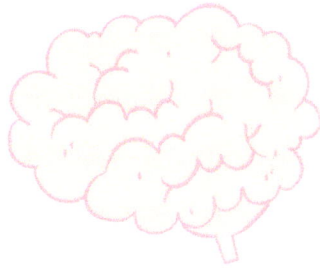

They help my BRAIN to be clever
so I can learn cool things forever.

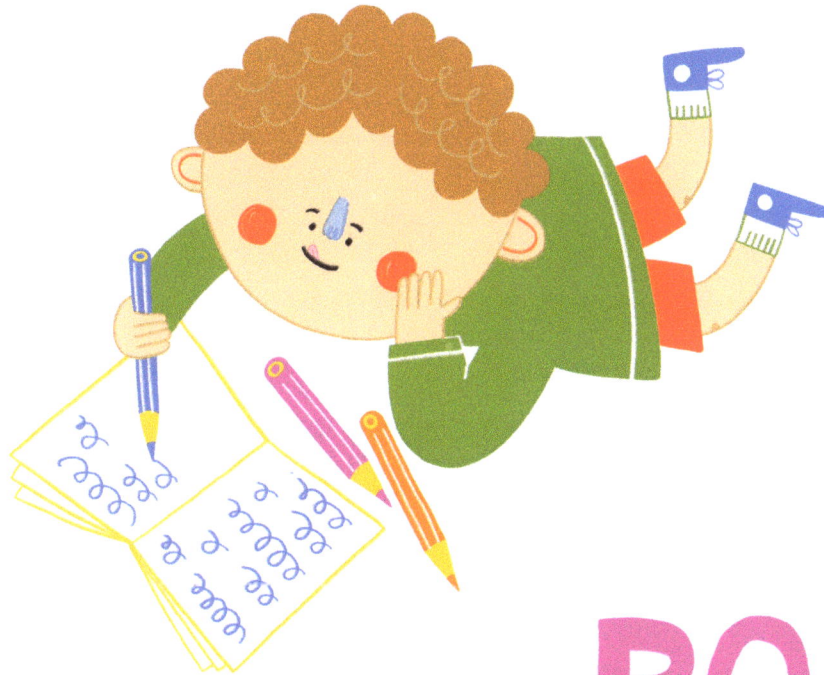

Then they come out as... **POO**.

My beetroot, pumpkin and lentils
go down into my tummy.

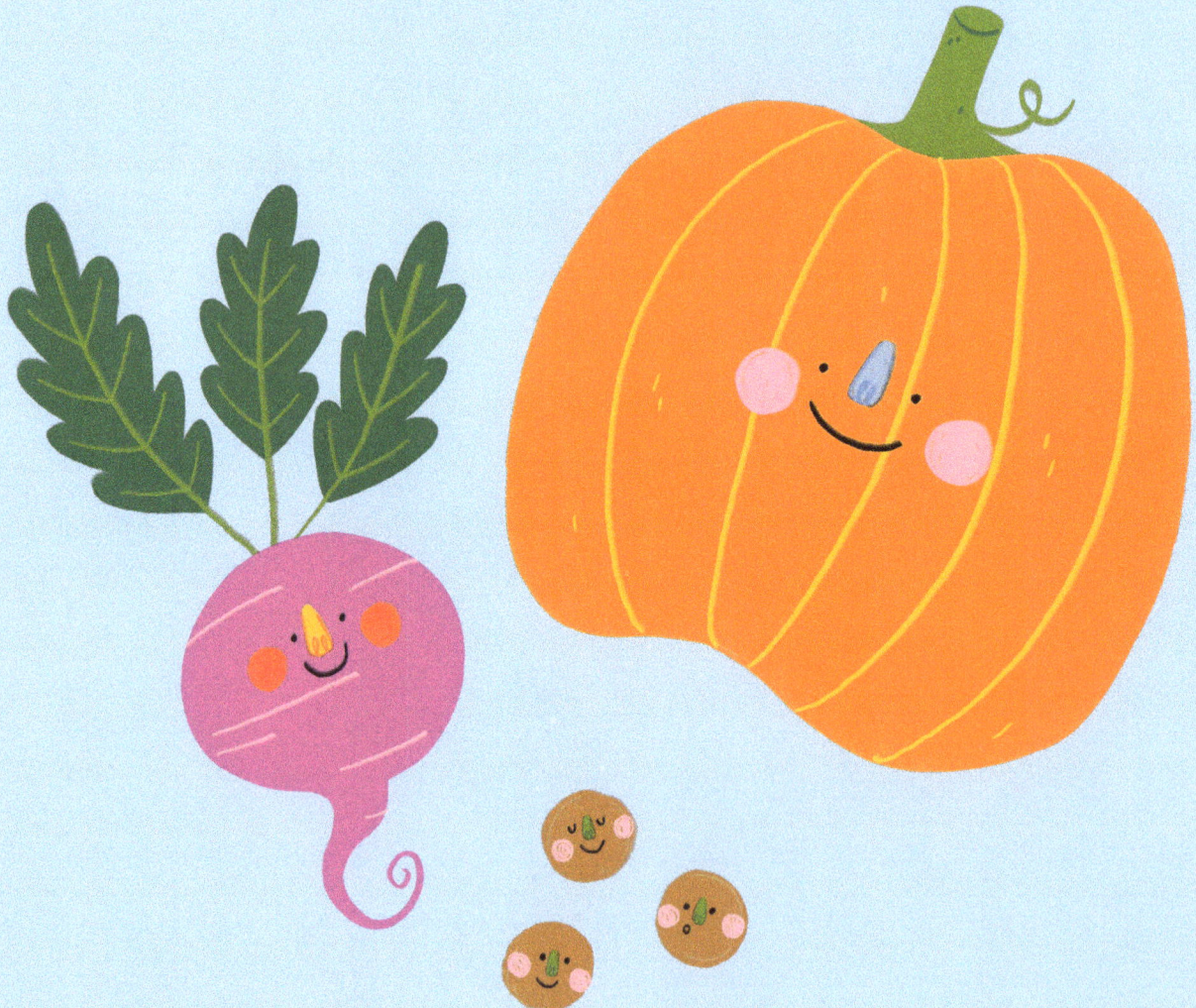

Then what do they do?

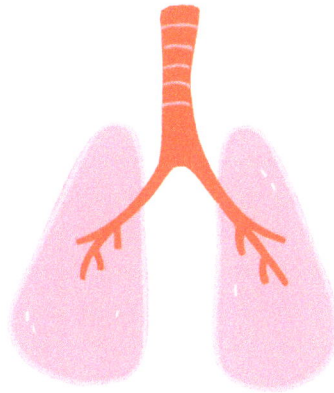

They help my LUNGS to fill with air
so I can sing without a care.

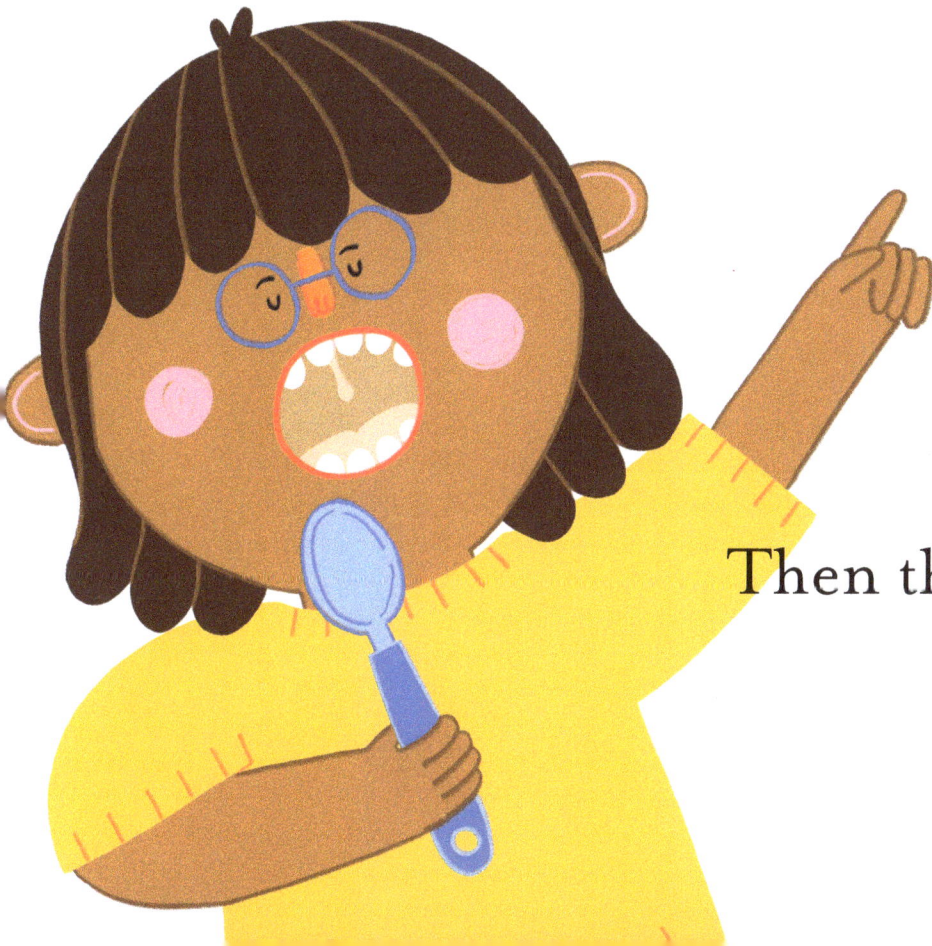

Then they come out as...

POO.

My cheese, milk and broccoli
go down into my tummy.

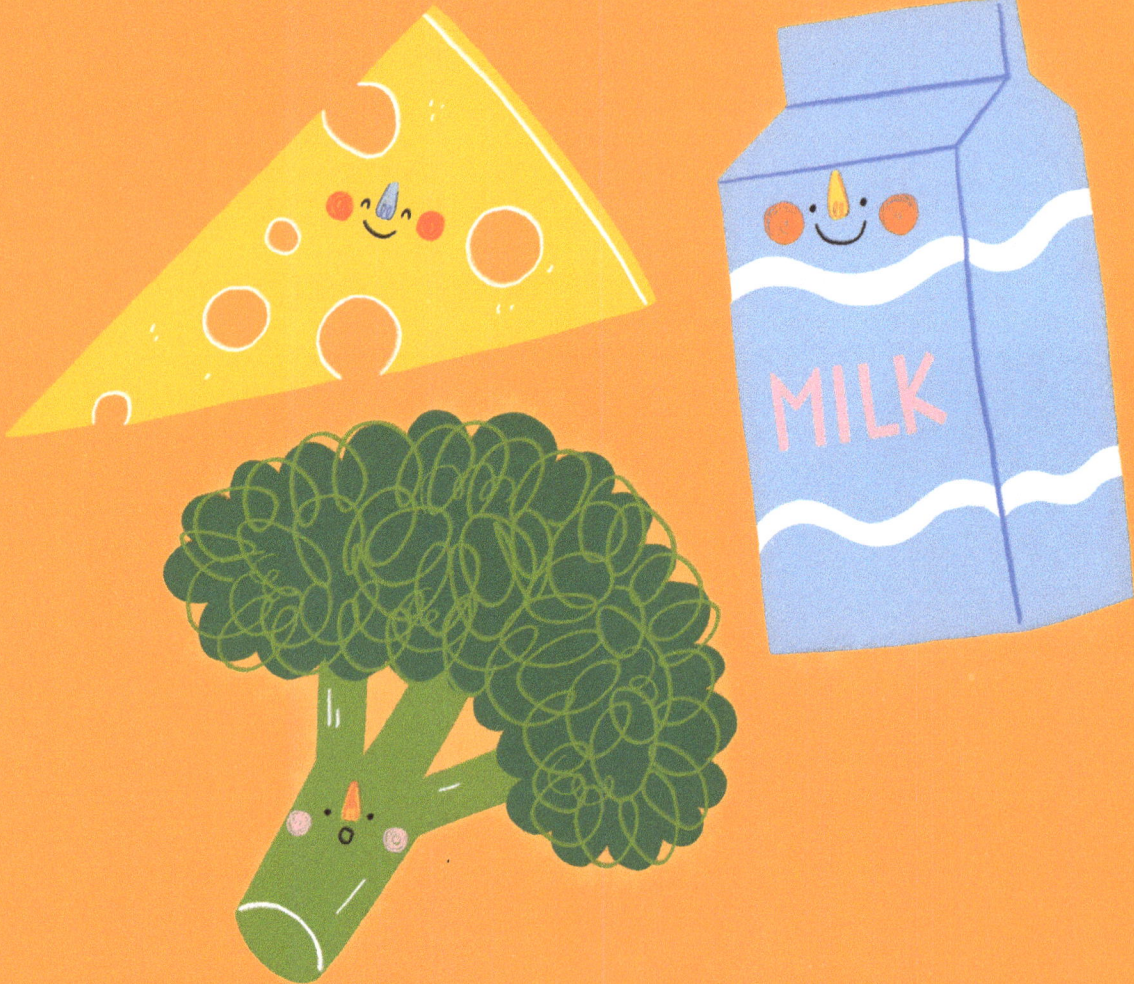

Then what do they do?

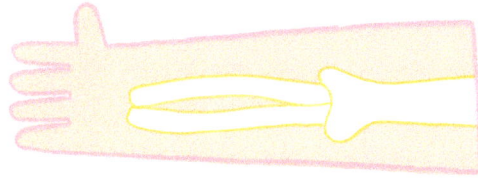

They help my BONES to grow strong and hard so I can play in my backyard.

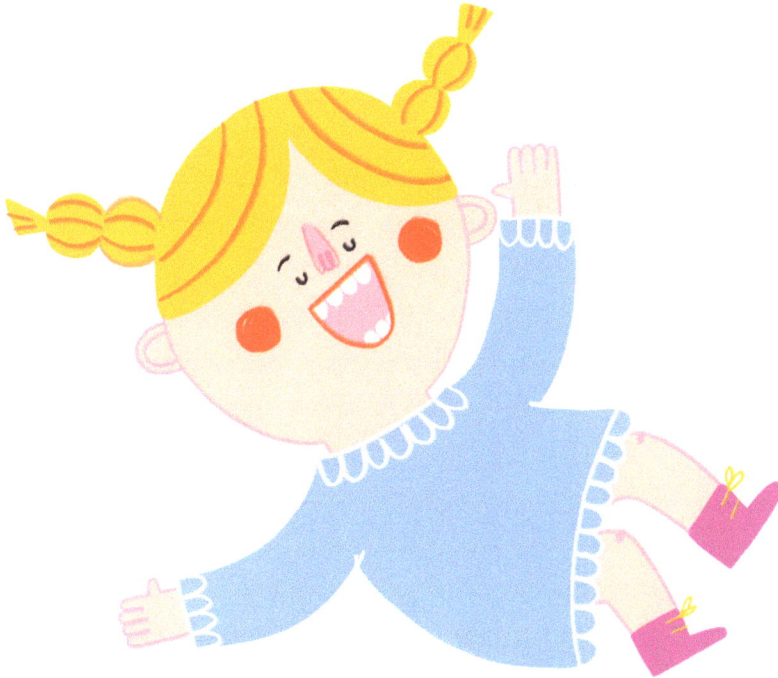

Then they come out as... POO.

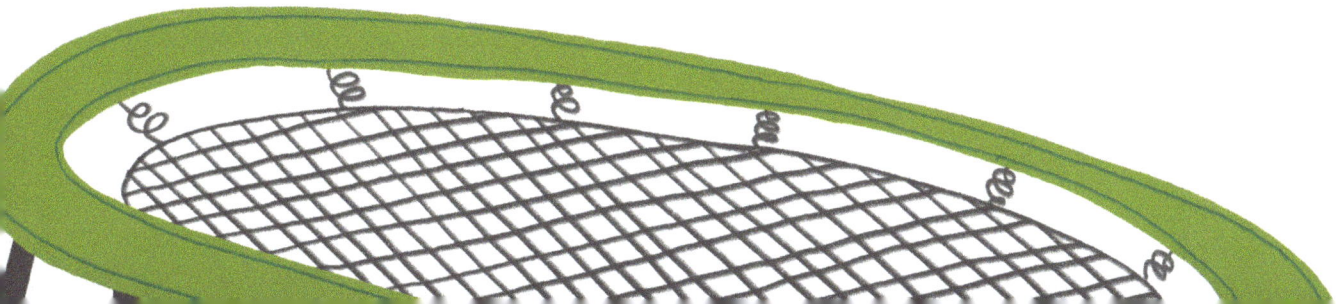

My egg, meat and beans
go down into my tummy.

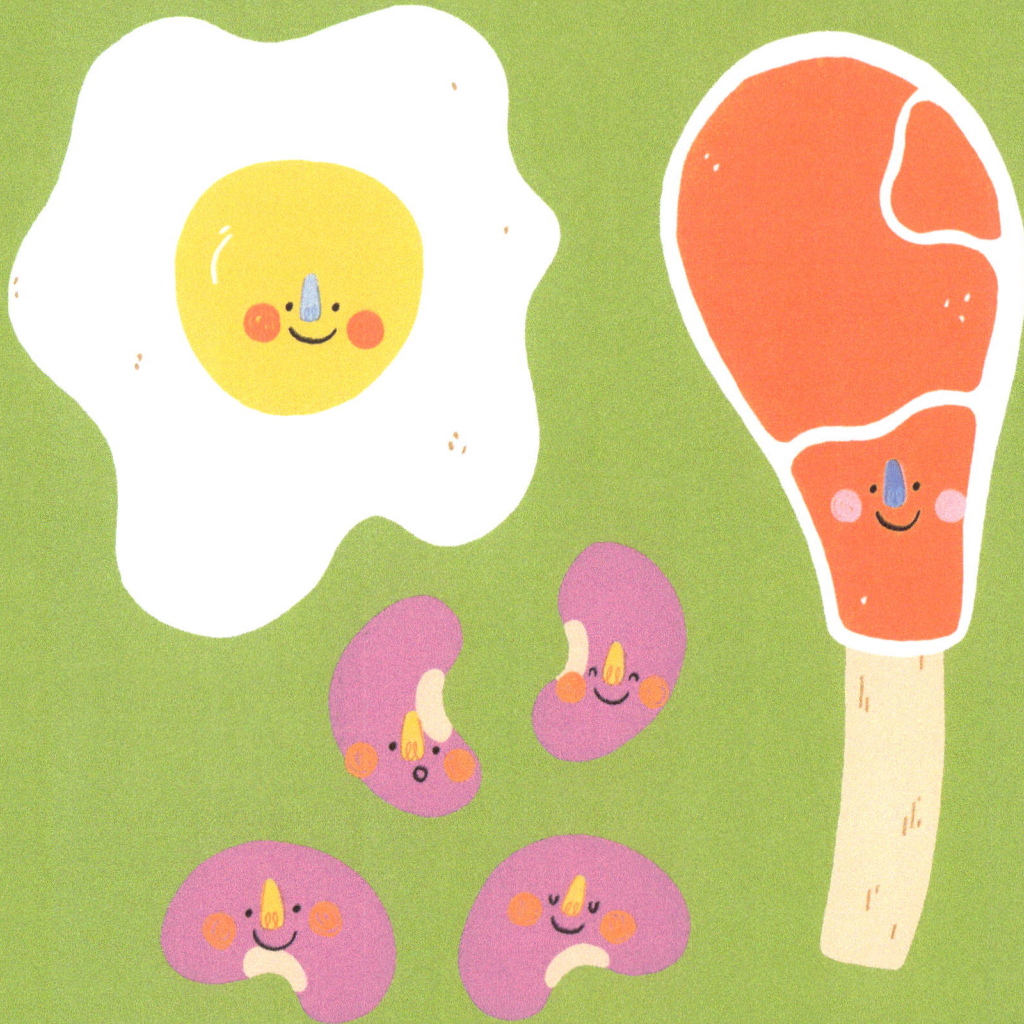

Then what do they do?

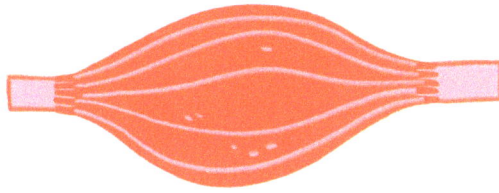

They help my MUSCLES get me moving
so I can keep on grooving.

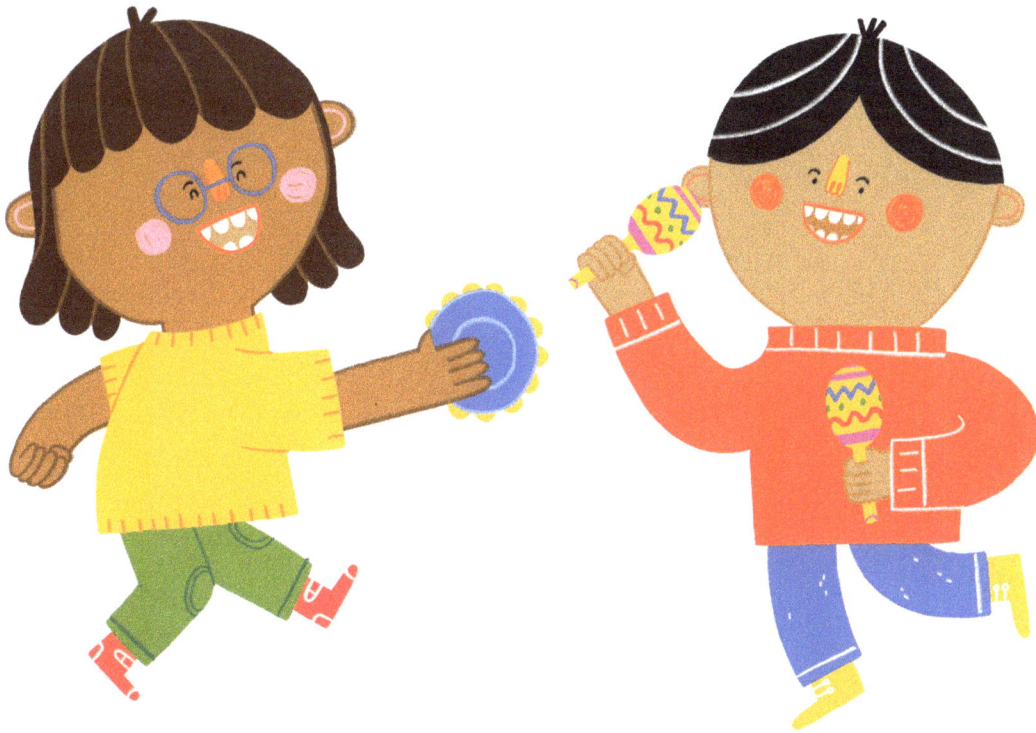

Then they come out as...

POO.

My carrot, peas and orange
go down into my tummy.

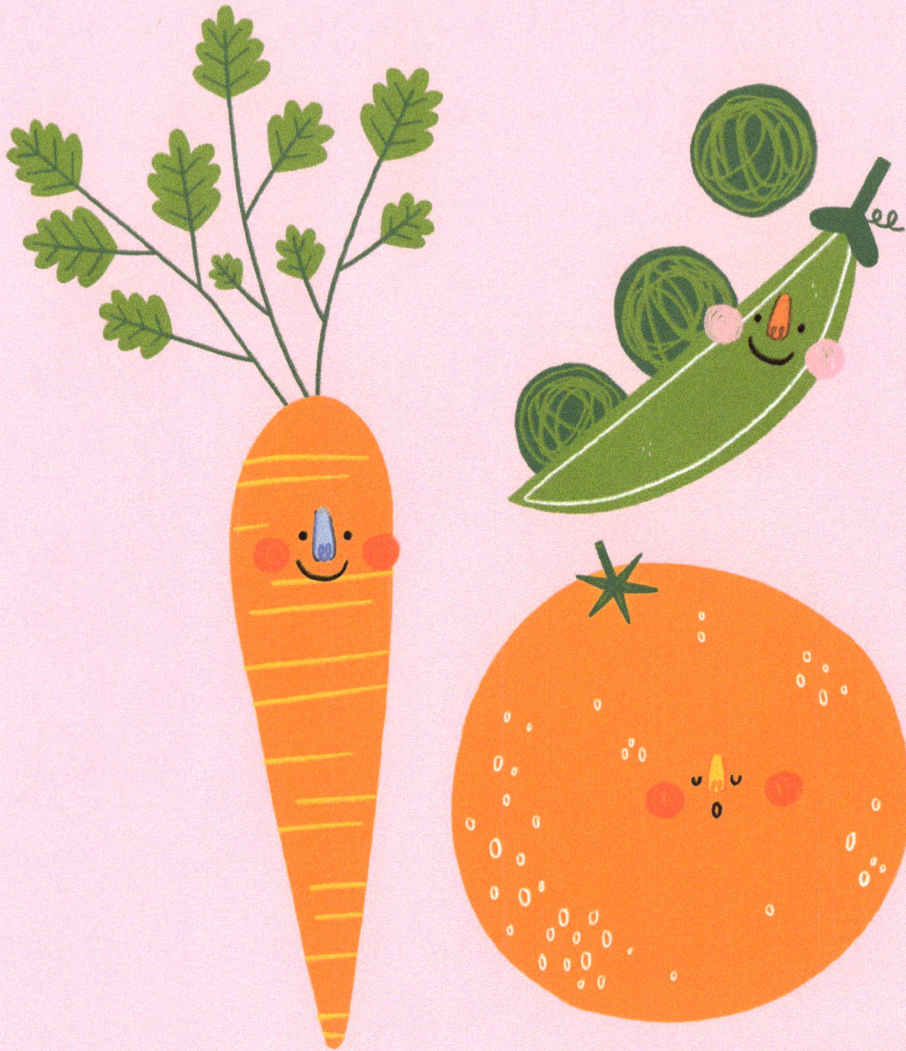

Then what do they do?

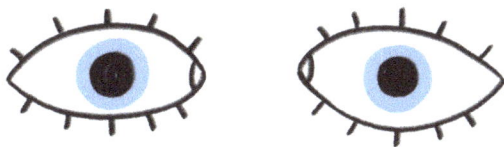

They help my EYES to open wide
so I can see the world outside.

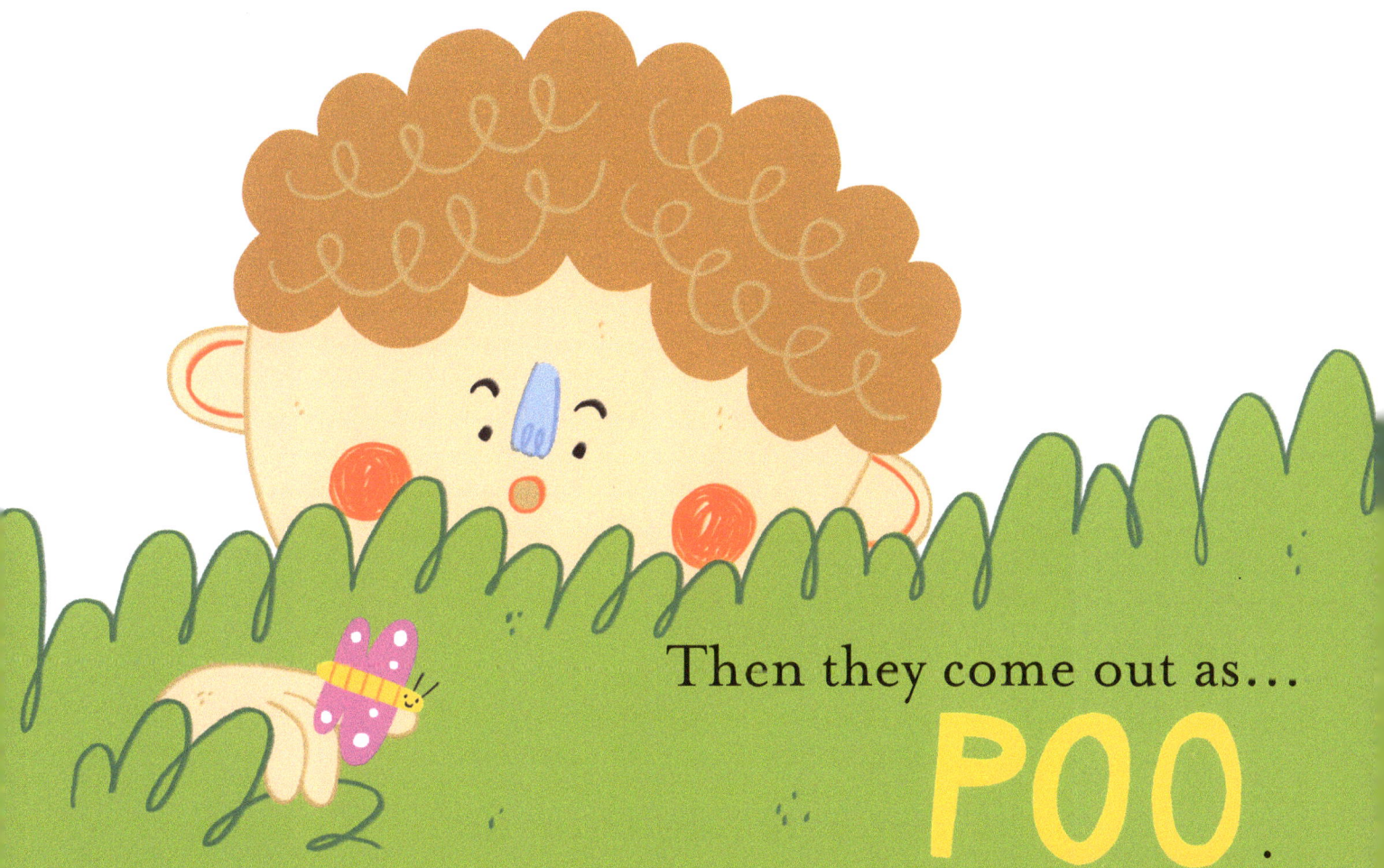

Then they come out as...
POO.

My tomato, grapes and sweet potato
go down into my tummy.

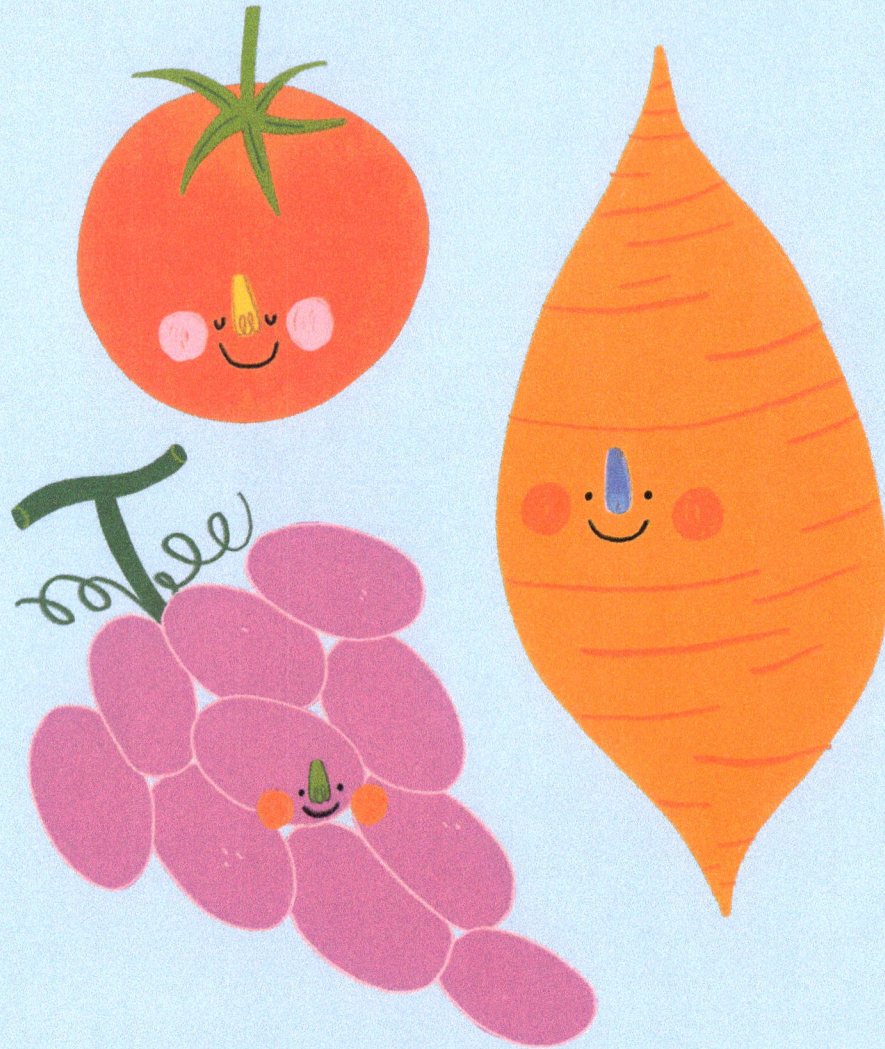

Then what do they do?

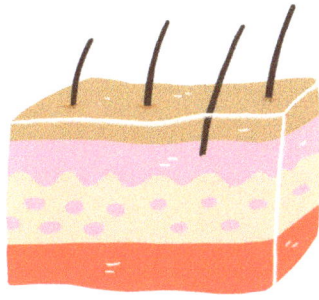

They help my SKIN to mend and heal
if I fall off my set of wheels.

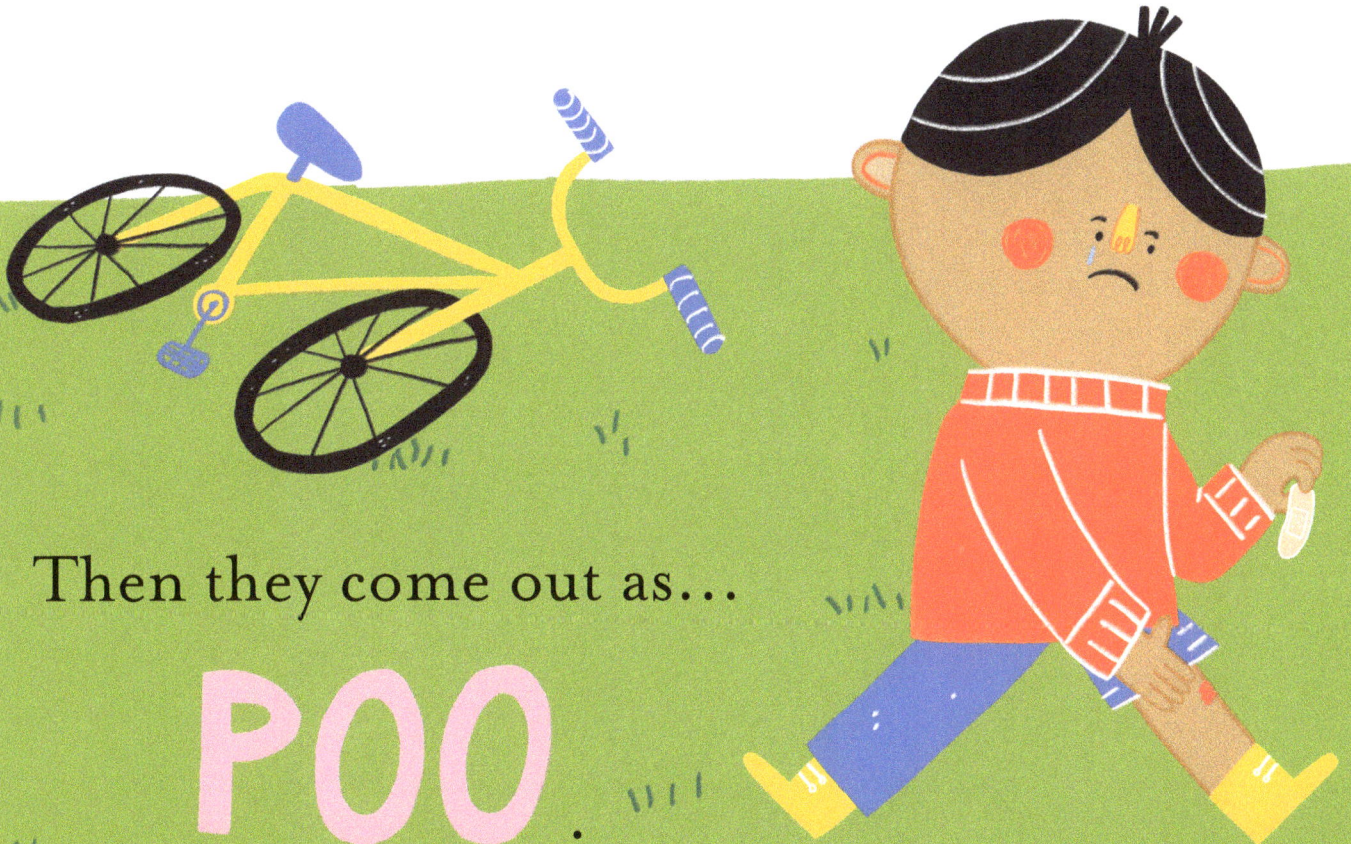

Then they come out as...

POO.

My apple, water and kiwi fruit
go down into my tummy.

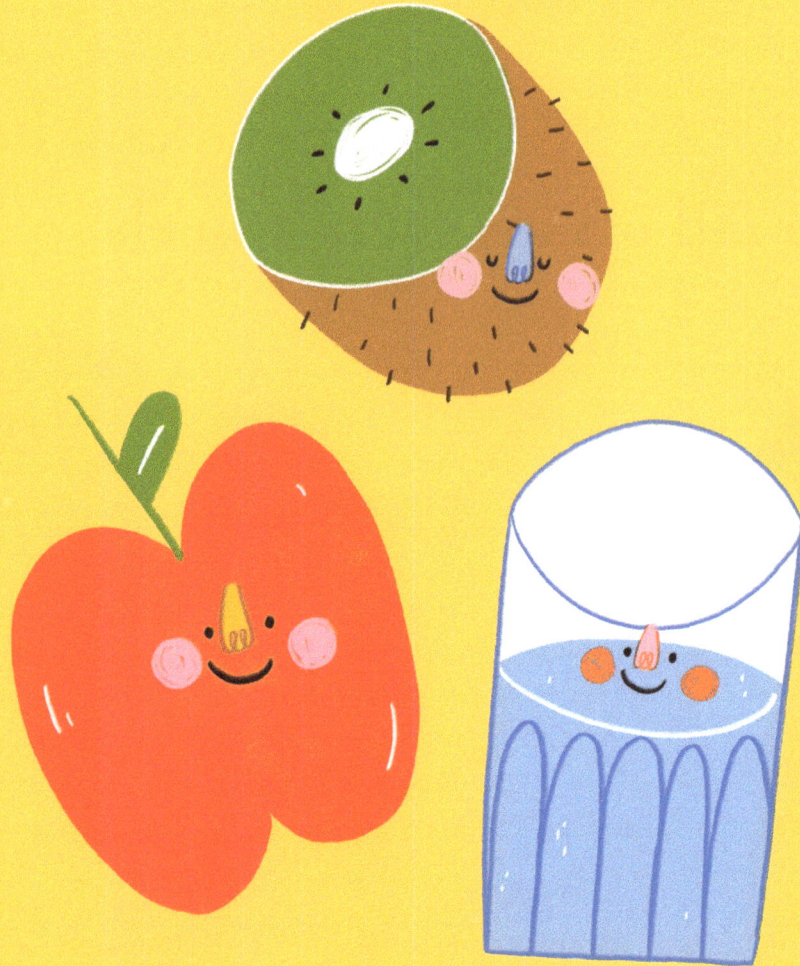

Then what do they do?

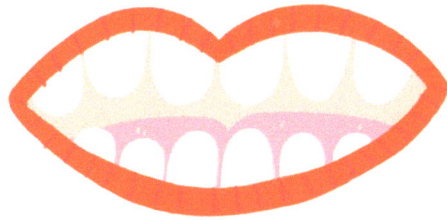

They help my TEETH stay strong and white
so I can chew and smile so bright.

Then they come out as…

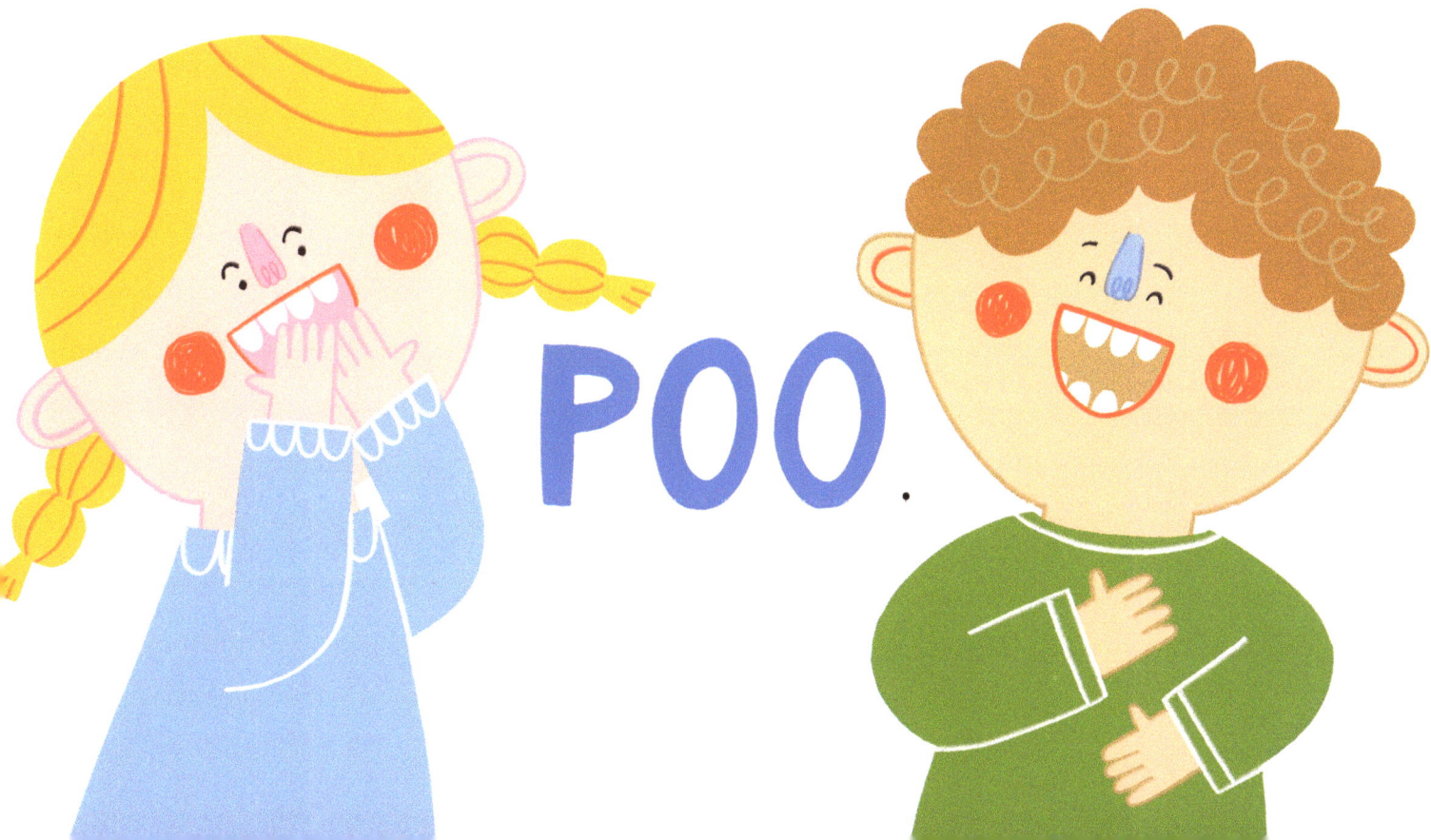

POO.

My yogurt, asparagus and banana
go down into my tummy.

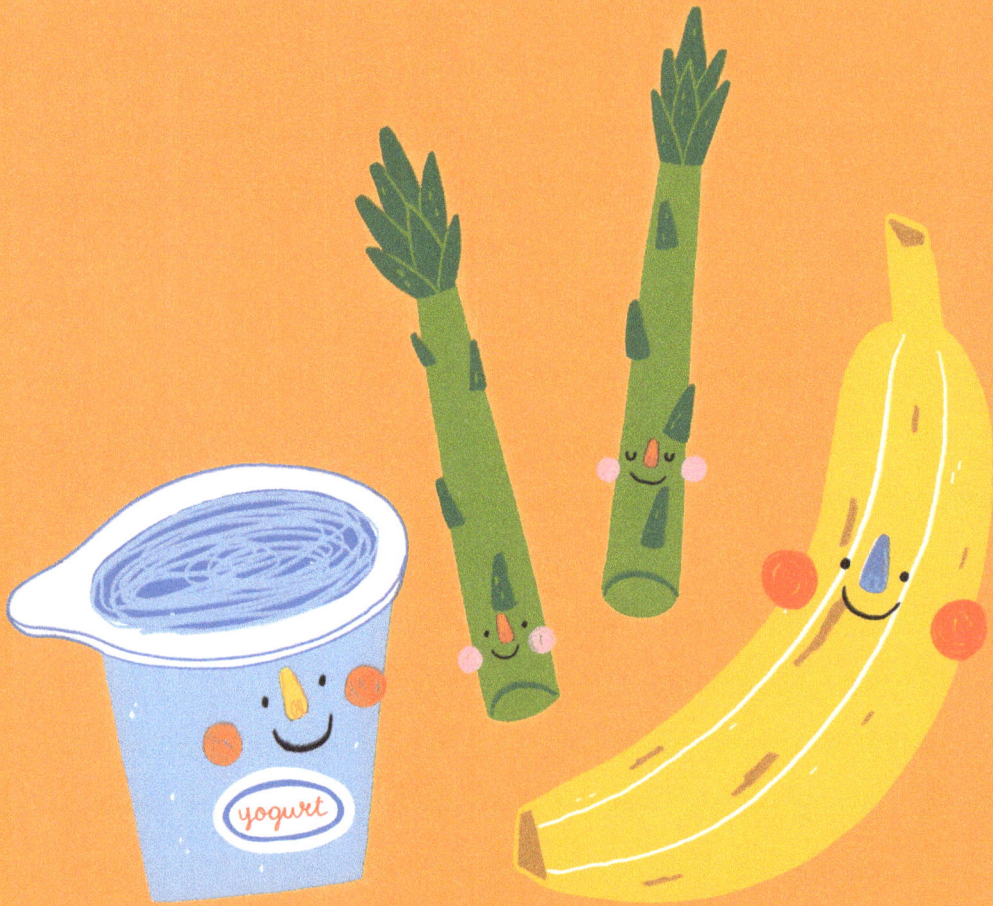

Then what do they do?

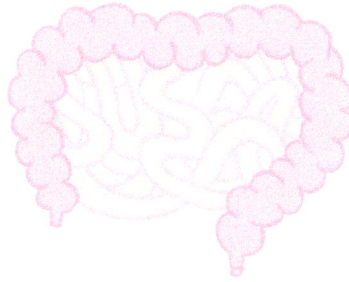

They help my INTESTINES digest food that I have bitten, munched and chewed.

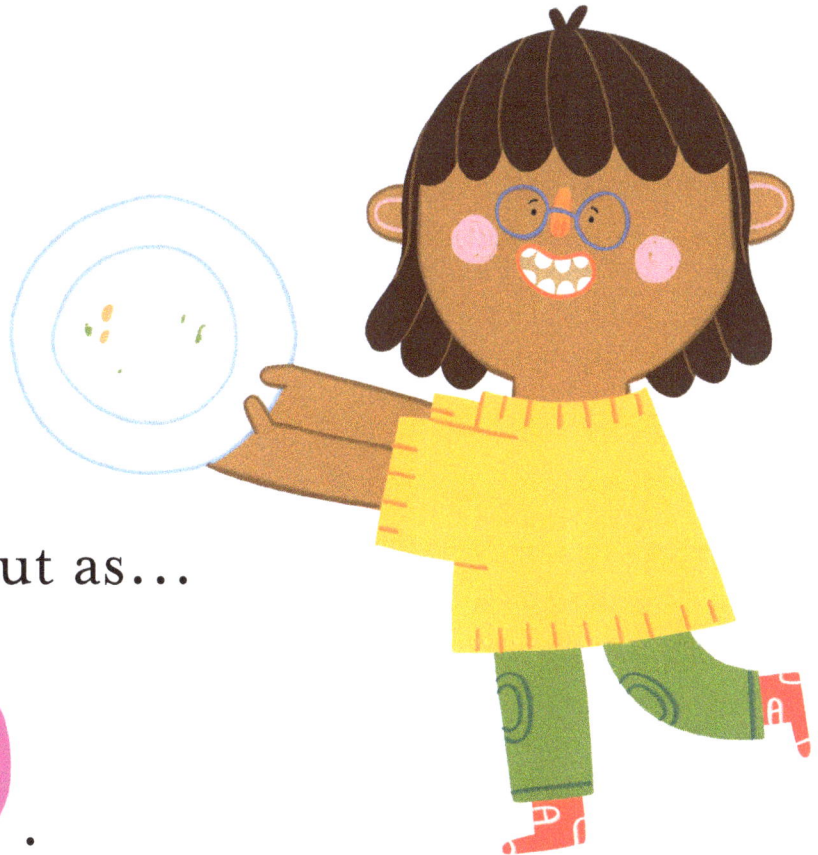

Then they come out as...

POO.

So when you swallow something yummy
down into your tummy…

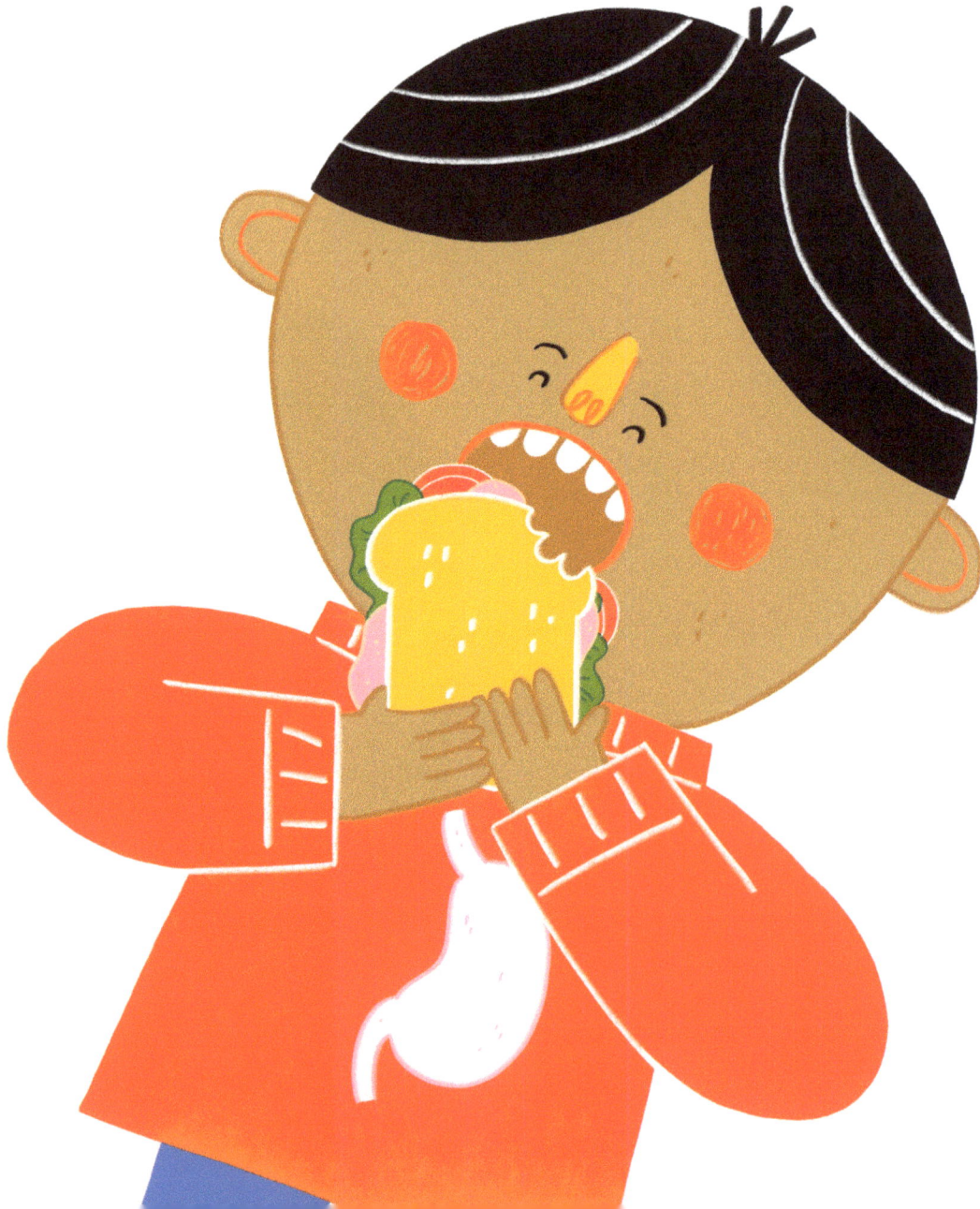

Remember your food works hard for you,

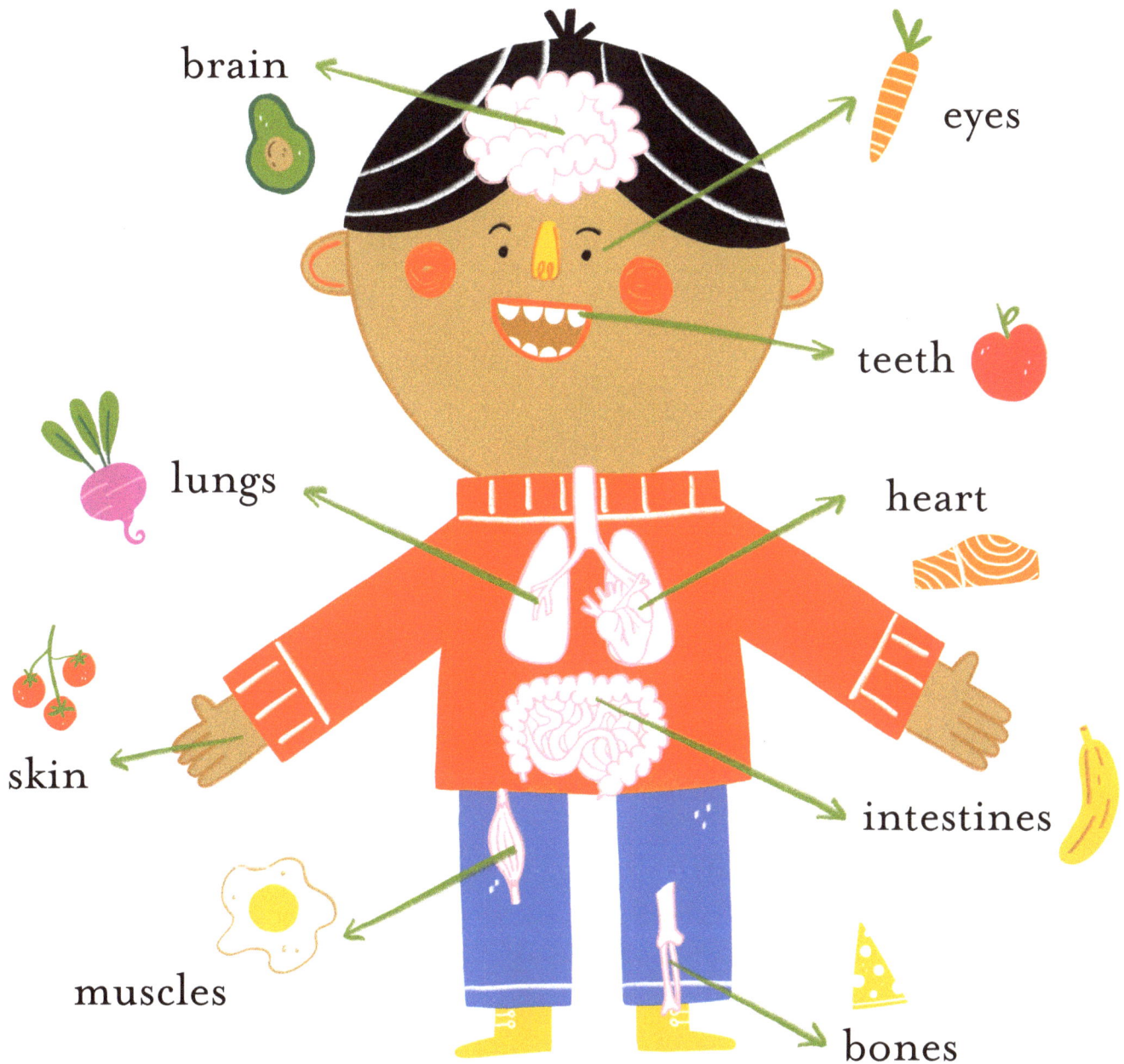

brain

eyes

teeth

lungs

heart

skin

intestines

muscles

bones

before it comes out as...

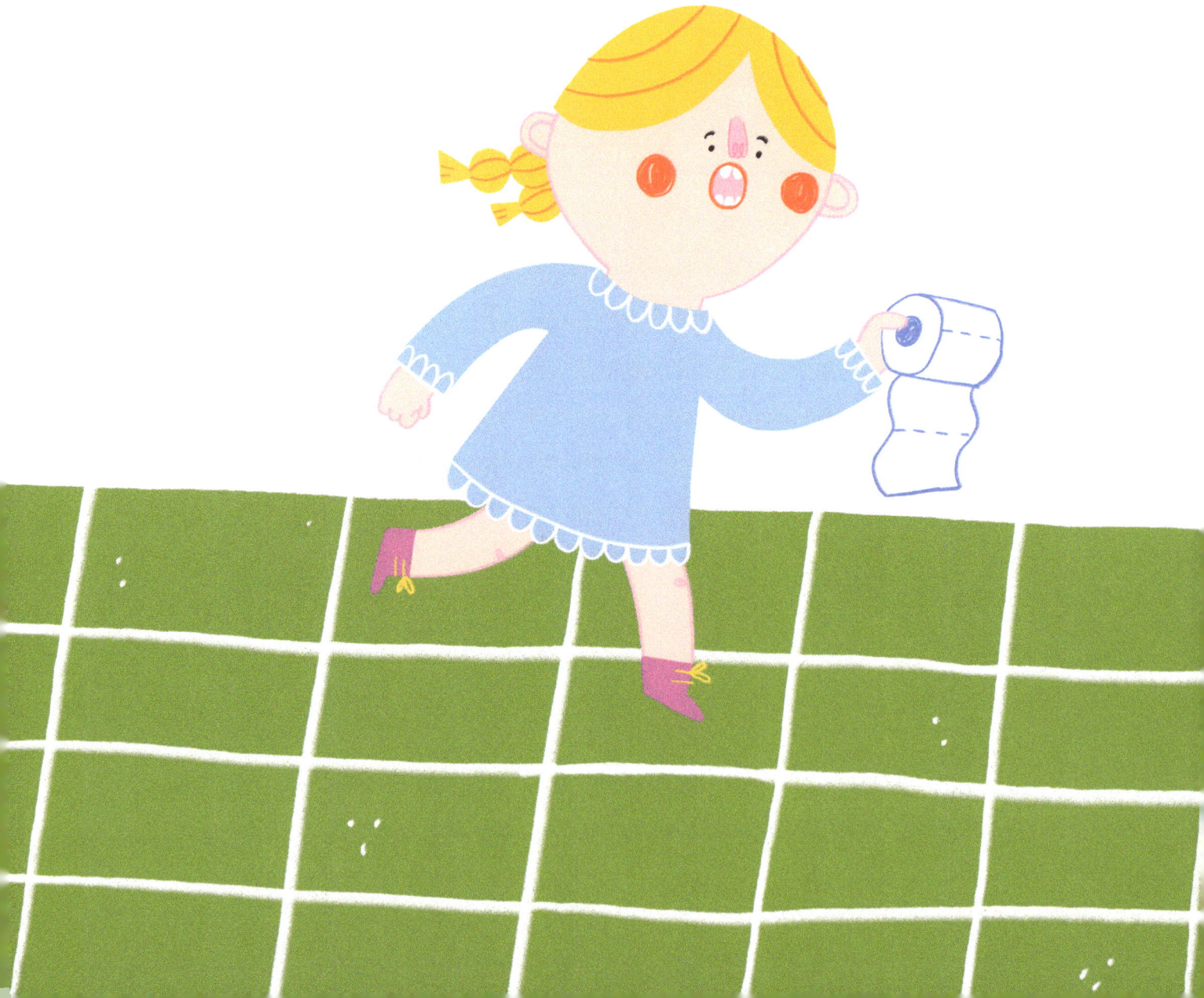

POO !

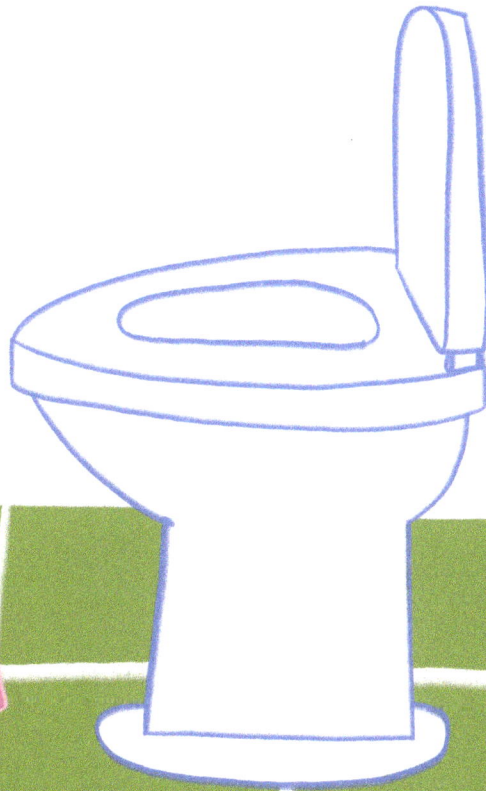
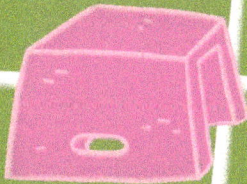

NOTES

for parents / grandparents / caregivers

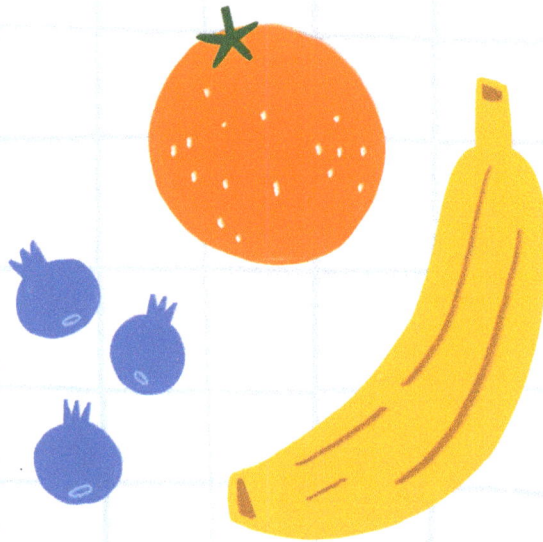

*Many of these foods contain a multitude of benefits which extend beyond the discussed organ and/or body function.

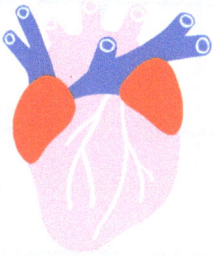

OATS contain a type of soluble fibre called beta-glucan which lowers blood glucose and cholesterol levels, thus helping to reduce the risk of heart disease and diabetes.

SALMON is rich in omega-3 fatty acids and potassium which help to reduce artery inflammation, lower cholesterol levels, and reduce the risk of heart disease.

SPINACH is a nutritional powerhouse packed with vitamins, minerals and fibre. It is particularly high in potassium and magnesium which help to relax blood vessels and lower blood pressure.

BLUEBERRIES are nutrient-dense and high in antioxidants and anthocyanidins which are believed to stimulate the flow of blood and oxygen to the brain and promote cognition and vascular health.

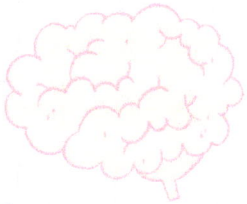

NUTS contain fatty acids, protein, vitamins, minerals and antioxidants which each play essential roles in many aspects of brain health including cognitive function, enhanced memory, learning and attention capacity.

AVOCADOS are full of essential nutrients and minerals which are required for brain growth and development, cell communication, cognition and psychological and neurological function.

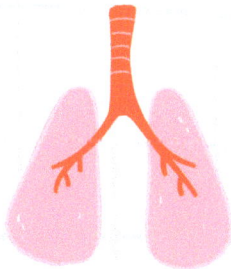

BEETROOT and beet greens (the leaves) are rich in nitrates which have been shown to benefit lung function and optimise oxygen intake.

PUMPKINS are especially rich in carotenoids which are associated with better lung function and have powerful antioxidant and anti-inflammatory properties.

LENTILS are part of the legume family and are high in nutrients that support lung function including magnesium, iron and potassium.

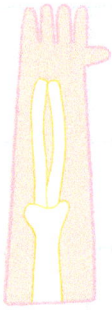

CHEESE is an excellent source of calcium and vitamin D, both essential for bone health. Adequate levels of calcium are also important for our teeth, heart, nerves, and muscles to function.

MILK is an excellent source of calcium, phosphorus and protein which are all important for bone health.

BROCCOLI is a good source of vitamin K and calcium, two vital nutrients for maintaining strong, healthy bones.

EGGS are rich in high-quality protein – supplying all 9 essential amino acids – and are therefore ideal for supporting muscle development, growth and repair.

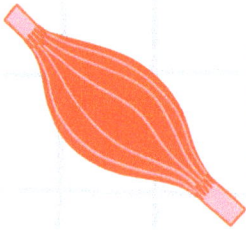

Red **MEAT** is an excellent source of protein, iron and zinc which are essential for muscle health, development and function. White meat is also a great source of lean protein which supports muscle growth and repair.

Part of the legume family, **BEANS** are rich in fibre and non-animal protein which help to keep us satisfied and build lean muscle mass.

CARROTS contain beta-carotene, a substance that the body converts to vitamin A which is an important nutrient for eye health.

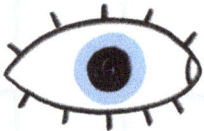

PEAS contain the carotenoids lutein and zeaxanthin which can help to protect our eyes from chronic diseases such as cataracts and age-related macular degeneration.

Citrus fruits like **ORANGES**, lemons and grapefruit are high in vitamin C which supports the health of blood vessels in the eyes.

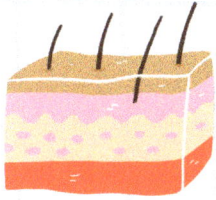

TOMATOES are an excellent source of vitamin C which can help stimulate collagen production and improve skin elasticity.

GRAPES contain an abundance of vitamin K, a nutrient which plays a critical role in blood clotting. Grapes are also high in enzymes which have anti-inflammatory effects and reparative functions for skin.

SWEET POTATOES are an excellent source of vitamin C which can help to boost collagen production which plays a role in skin elasticity and strength.

Chewing an **APPLE** stimulates saliva production which helps to rinse food particles and bacteria away from our teeth. Additionally, the vitamins and minerals found in apples such as vitamin C and potassium, contribute to gum health.

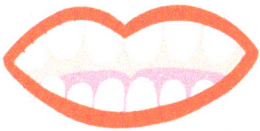

KIWI FRUITS contain high levels of vitamin C which strengthens gums and helps protect against gum inflammation called gingivitis. Kiwis are also packed full of calcium which helps to neutralise acids while boosting enamel health.

Acids from plaque, food, and other drinks can harm our tooth enamel and attract cavity-causing bacteria. Drinking **WATER** dilutes these acids, helping to fight against cavities, gum disease and protect tooth enamel.

YOGURT that is high in protein, calcium, vitamins, live cultures and probiotics can enhance gut health and digestion.

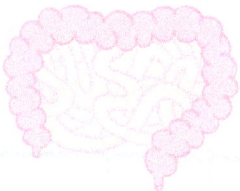

The dietary fibre in **ASPARAGUS** promotes good bacteria which helps our stomach and intestines to digest our food and absorb important nutrients.

BANANAS are high in a type of soluble fibre called pectin, which helps with digestion through regulating bowel movements and supporting the growth of good bacteria in the digestive tract.

www.ingramcontent.com/pod-product-compliance
Lightning Source LLC
Chambersburg PA
CBHW041608260326
41914CB00012B/1428

This book has been given with love to

_____

from

_____,
your relationship

_____.
your name(s)

_____

_____

_____

Home Is a Feeling

Of Course I Want to Be Home

Written and Illustrated by Mary Beth Husman
Designed to Be Worthy 2022

Published by:
Designed to Be Worthy
102 W.McElhaney Road
Taylors, SC 29687

© 2022, Designed to Be Worthy
ISBN: 978-1-7923-8054-9

No part of this book is to be copied,
transmitted, stored, or otherwise taken
without express written consent.

Dedication

    I dedicate this book to my mother, Sally Mae (Keiper) Tompkins, who has taught me so much in life and who continues to teach me from her new home in Memory Care. I thank you for the example you are. I love you, Mom. My heart is with you in this journey. You bless me and my family beyond measure.

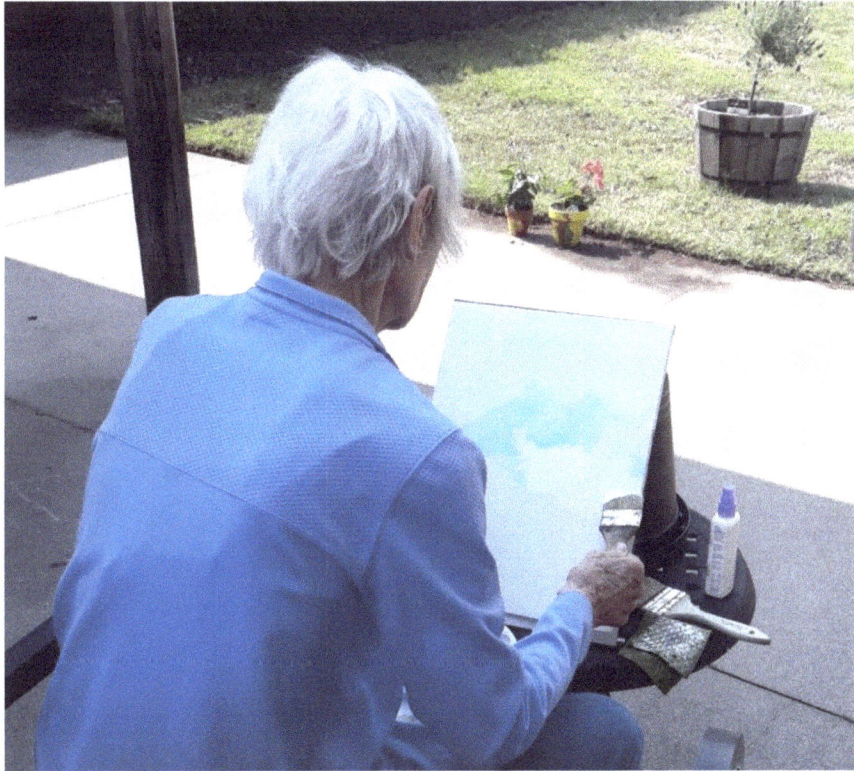

(Sally moved to her new home in Glory, August 24, 2022.)

Foreword

"I want to go home." Of course! This is a true feeling. We all want to feel at home. We want to be in a familiar place with a familiar routine and in connection with people we know.

This book shines a new light on this longing for home. Browsing the pages, engaging in its soft, colorful paintings, enjoying the repetitive beginning to each new page spread, and reading the few but gentle words below each image molds this longing into a positive reflection on the here and now. This little book provides gentle reassurance that the feelings of being comfortably at home can be found in the little, everyday moments.

Uncluttered pages, large and bold text, and short phrases provide the opportunity to continue the pastime of reading even when sight or long texts are frustrations. Importantly, the format of this book encourages meaningful, shared moments of conversation between readers. So, cuddle up with this book or sit side by side with your loved one and enjoy the moment.

Feel joy. Be still. And be at peace.

Dear one,

I hear you! I hear your heart.

Let's share the pages of this book.

Together, we will find the peace,

comfort, and contentment

of home.

Home is a feeling. . .

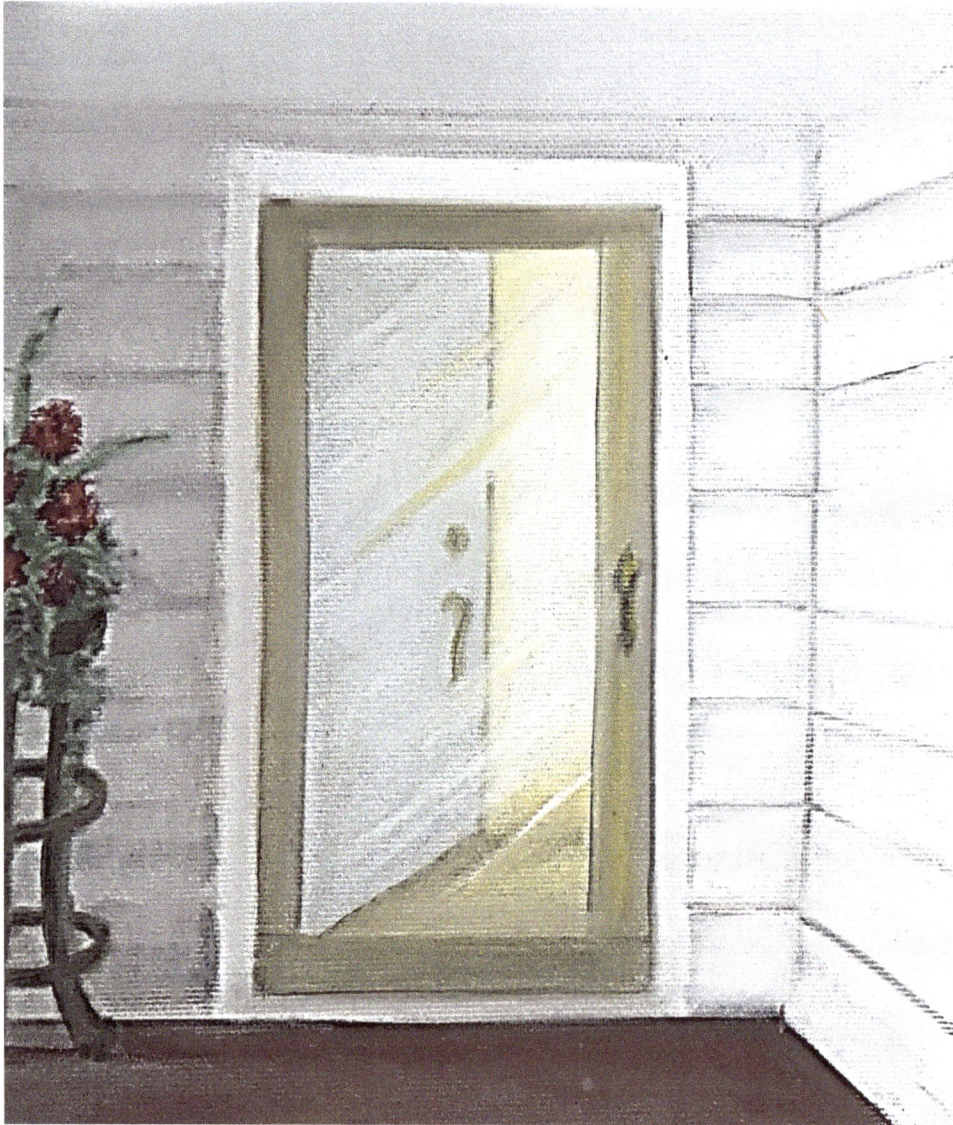

of belonging somewhere familiar.

hearing that special little knock at the door

seeing a familiar and joyful smile

rocking in the front porch rocker

smelling home-baked cookies

being wrapped in a tender hug

settling down into a favorite chair

cozying under a soft lap blanket

resting your head gently on your pillow

Home is a feeling . . .

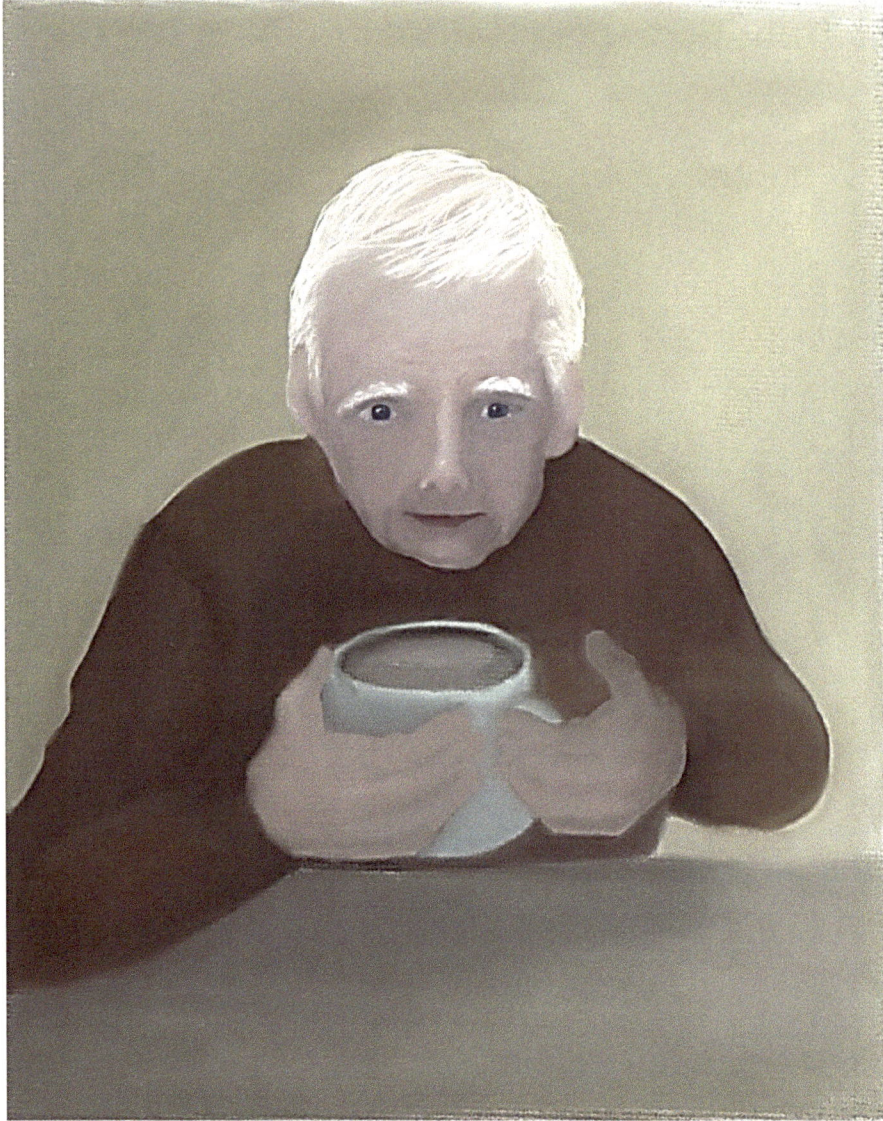

of being sure of the routine.

starting the day with a warm drink to sip

dressing for the day

morning prayers and reading

listening to television

tidying up little messes

going for a walk

talking on the phone

cooking in the kitchen

tucking into bed at night

Home is a feeling . . .

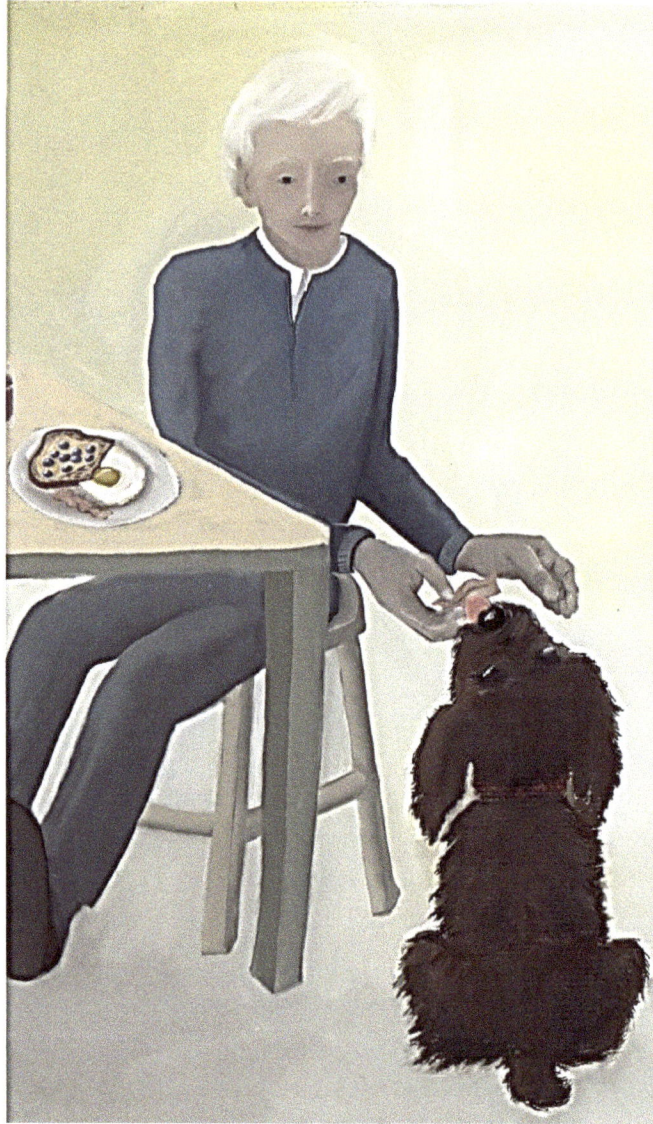

of caring for others.

a soft, furry pet

a loved one

family

friends

neighbors

a precious child

a stranger in need

Home is a feeling . . .

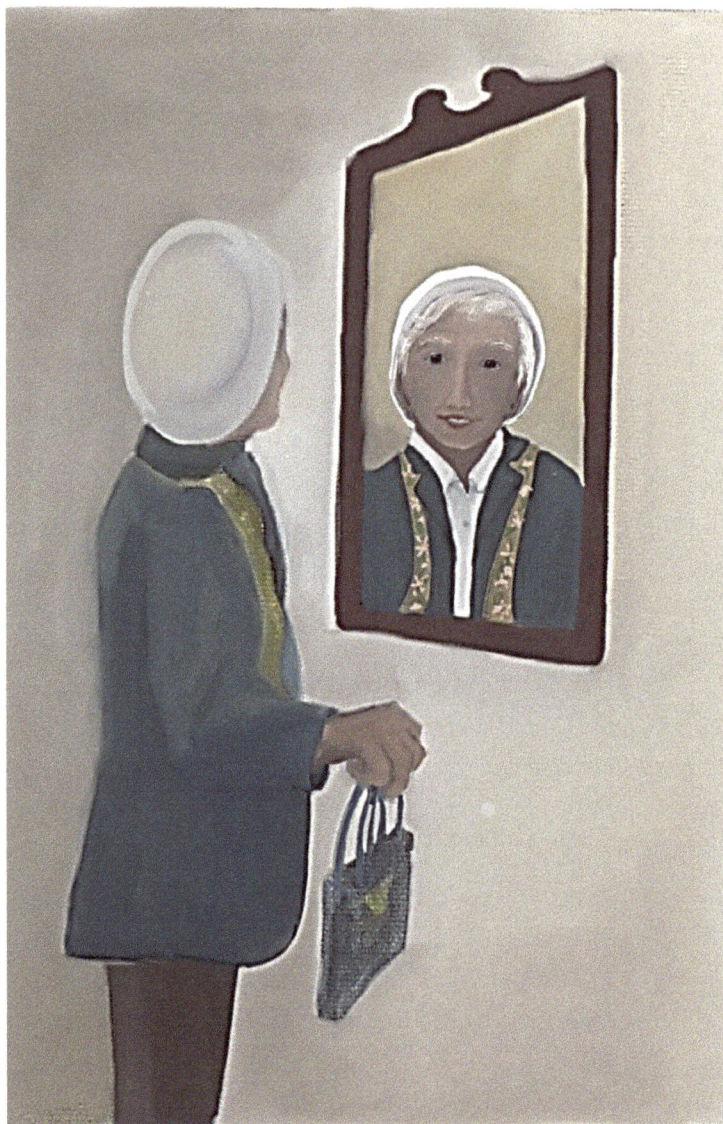

of keeping up with time.

places to go

people to see

things to do

appointments to keep

blessings to give

meals to eat

praises to sing

Home is a feeling . . .

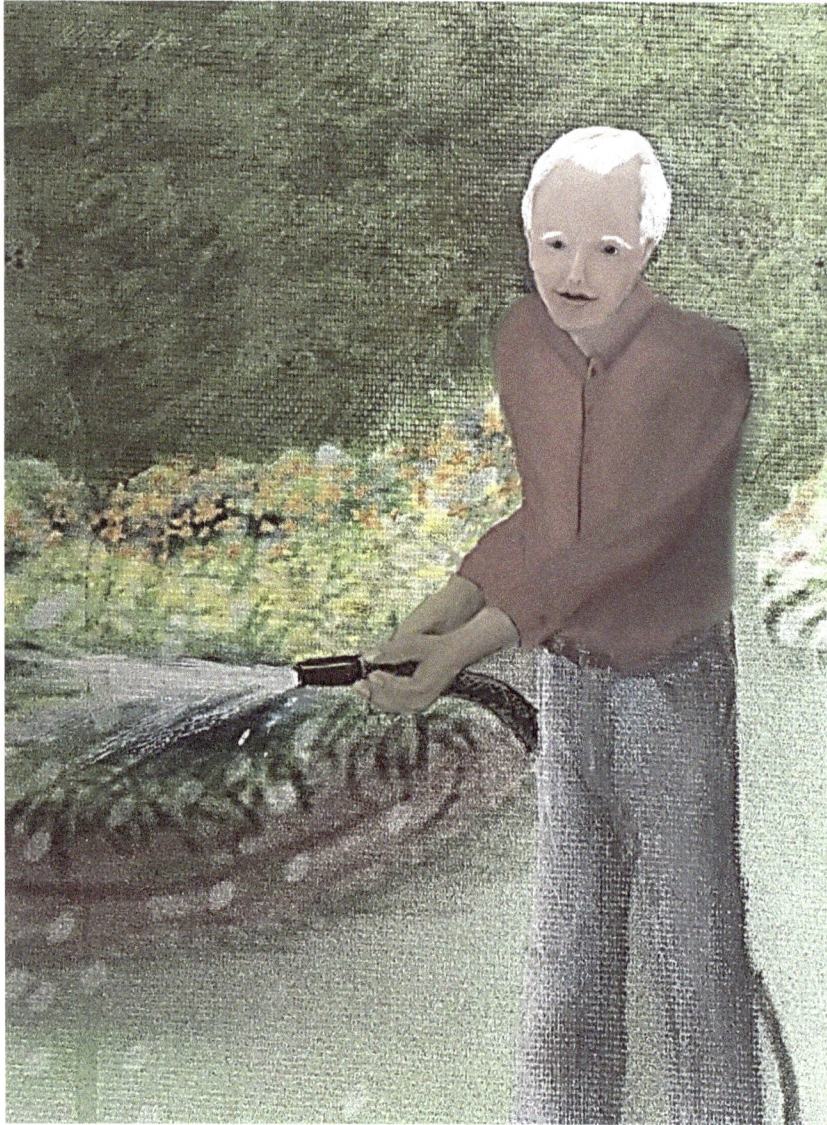

of finding delight in a place.

watering in the garden

rocking on the porch

cooking in the kitchen

working at your project table

tending clothes in the laundry

talking on the telephone in a cozy chair

Home is a feeling . . .

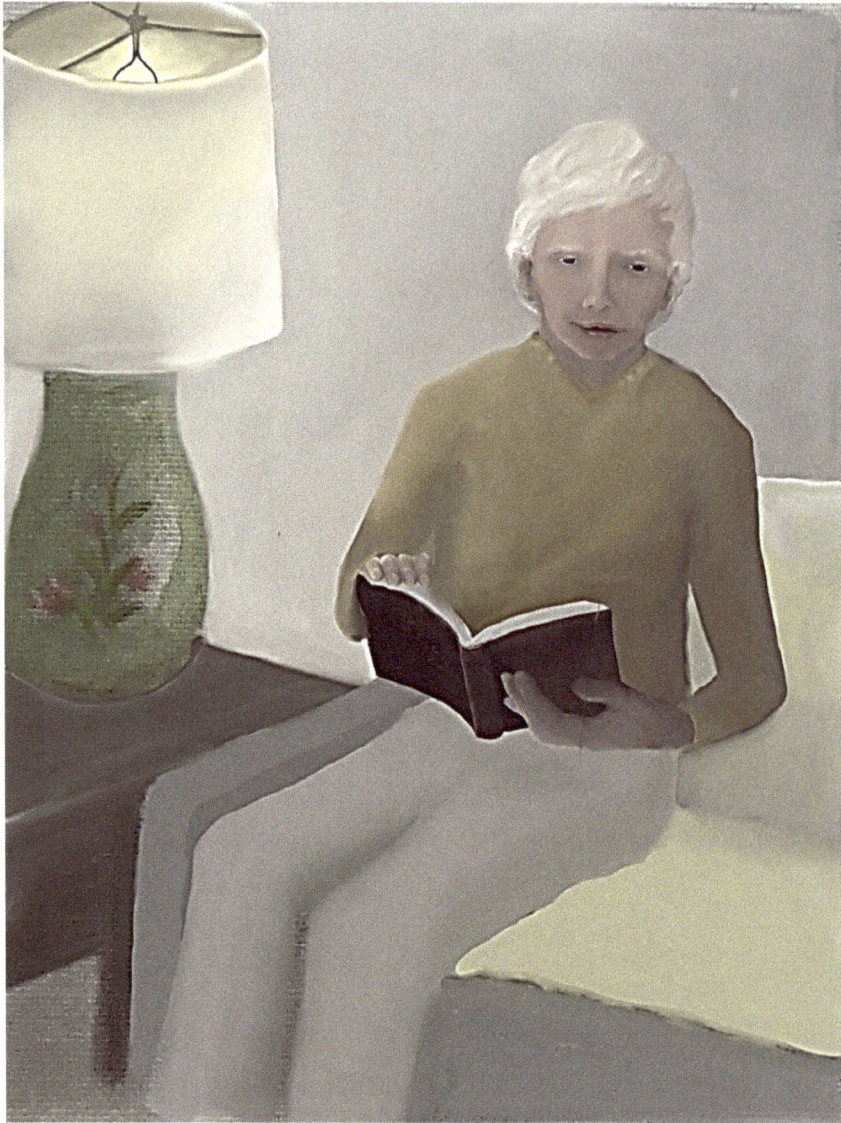

of passing time peacefully.

reading a book

visiting with a friend

taking a nap

writing letters

watching a bird outside

enjoying music

caressing a pet

Home is a feeling . . .

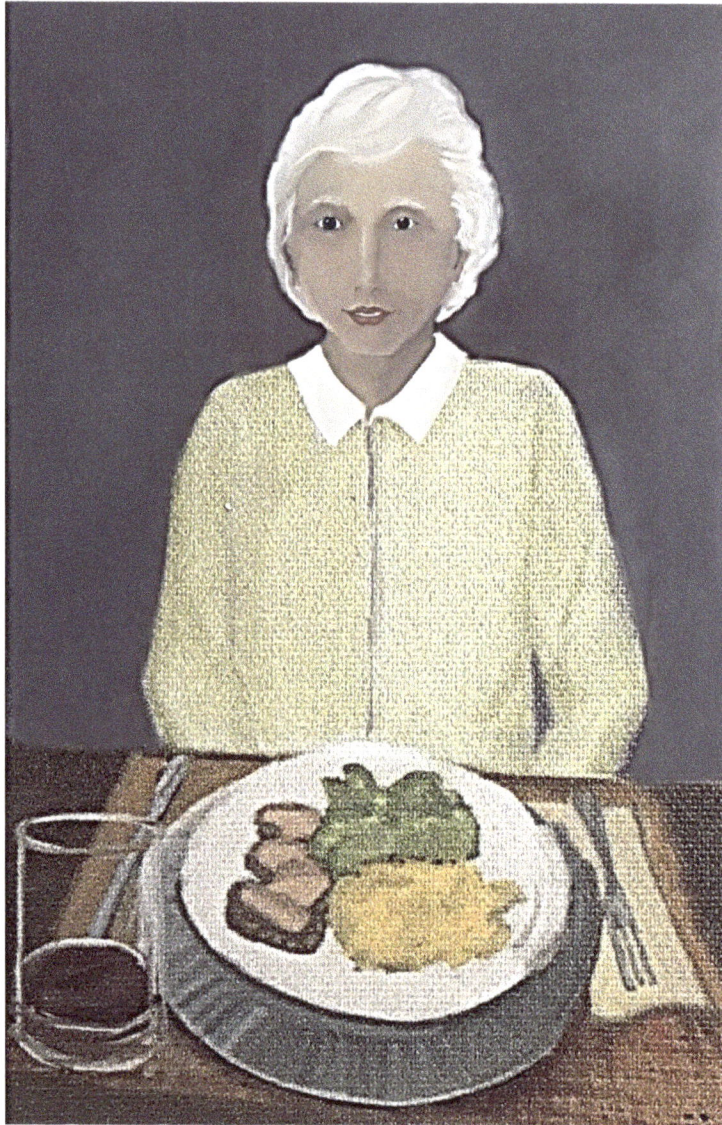

of enjoying a warm meal.

savoring favorite foods

sipping a sweet tea

lingering in conversation

tasting a beautiful dessert

having a full belly

Home is a feeling . . .

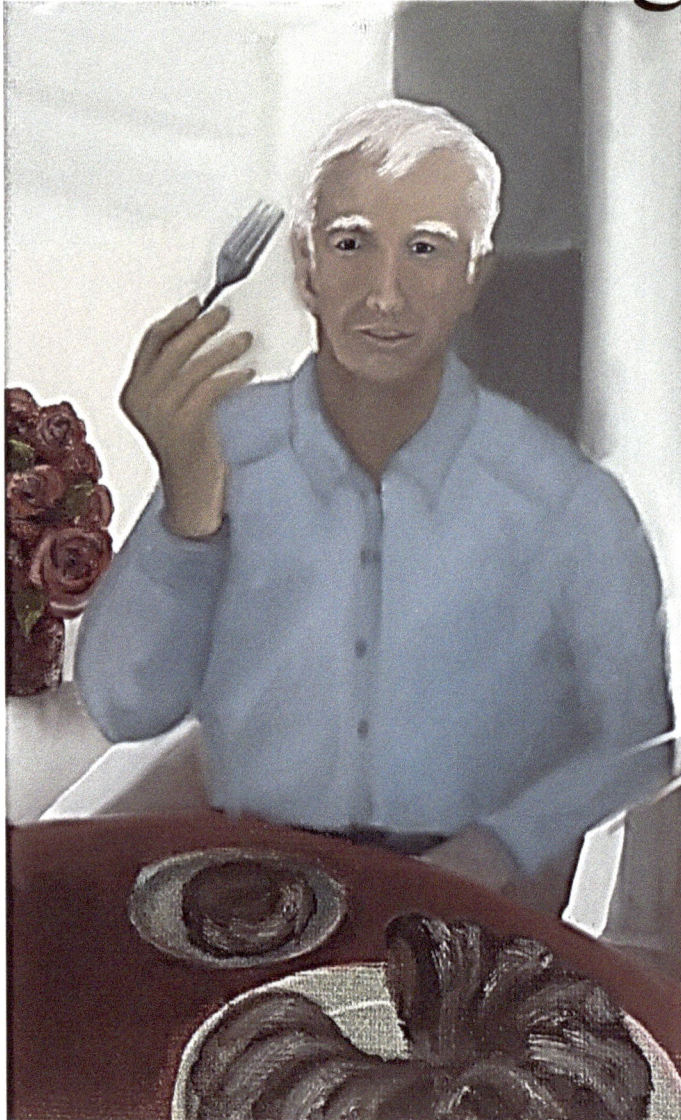

of celebrating.

a birthday

a holiday

an accomplishment

a special day

an ordinary day

simply nothing at all

the taste of sweetness

Home is a feeling . . .

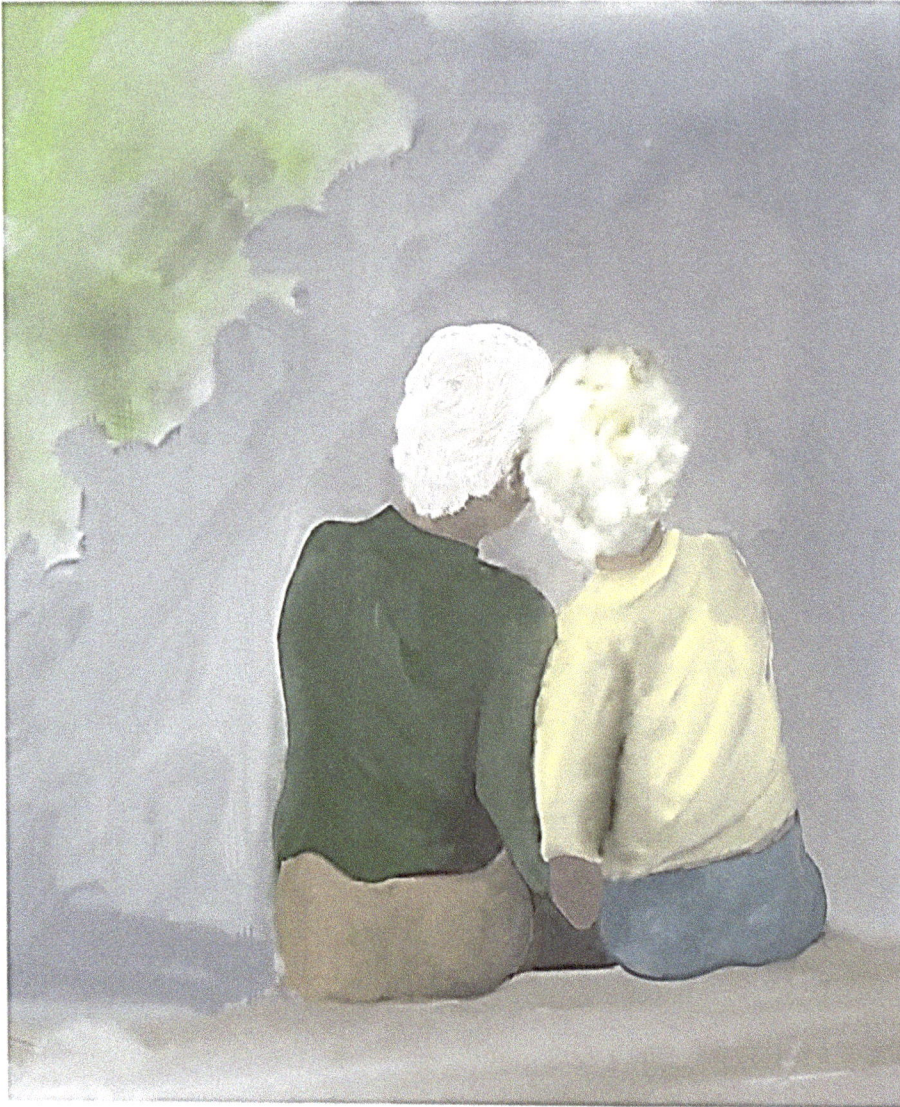

of connecting to a familiar heart song.

Jesus hears your heart song.

[2] "In my Father's house are many mansions . . .
I go to prepare a *Home* for you . . .

[3] I will come again, and receive you unto myself;
that where I am, there you may be also."

You know the way:
[6] "I am the way, the truth, and the life…"

His invitation to you: *Come to the Father by me.*

John 14:2-6.
Italicized text is a paraphrase for clarity.

Home is a feeling . . .

of comfort, love, and peace.

Dear precious Father in heaven,

I am blessed to be your child, and I put my trust

in your saving Grace. Please forgive my wrongs.

Hold my hand securely as I walk with You.

Comfort me in your loving embrace.

Give me your peace and allow me to rest

in your goodness. I belong here.

I am at Home in you.

Through Christ Jesus I pray these things,

Amen.

About the Author

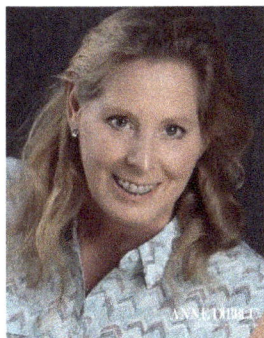

Mary Beth Husman lives in Greenville, South Carolina. She is wrapped in hugs from her loving husband, her son and his precious wife, three lively grandchildren, memories of her daughter, her brother and his family, her sister and her family, and a host of cherished friends.

As of the writing of this book, she also is blessed to lavish much time on her mom Sally, to whom this book is dedicated, and her dad, Dale, who now lives with the Husmans in his own special quarters recently built just for him. Dale still enjoys frequent trips to spend time with the love of his life, and Sally enjoys visitors!

Although this is her first illustrated book available to anyone outside of family, the author has been in love with words and art for a very long time, since childhood. Artistic inclinations from her mother together with a mind for engineering from her dad were foundational to her thirty year career as a graduate landscape architect, a blend of art, engineering, and plants. Mary Beth enjoyed home educating their two children until they left for university, and then she spent the next ten years leading an Art FUNdamentals class and four levels of English composition (with grammar, vocabulary, and literature) at a local home school co-op.

After ten years of leading students, Mary Beth planned for retirement at the end of the school year. She needed to spend more time helping her father and mother. By spring, her mother had begun her journey in earnest while no one was looking. In a matter of a few months, they needed to move from their home to a place where each of them had the care they needed. An unseen difficulty arose between the time of application to the new community and the mid-December 2020 actual move: because of COVID new residents were required two weeks of forced quarantine from outside visitors, family, that is. Sally was already confused about her new home, but to suddenly be without her husband, her house, and her dog was unusually cruel. It is from these experiences that this book came into being. Mom needed comfort. She needed to feel at home. And, many families make this same journey and their family member also needs comfort and to feel at home.

At: https://designedtobeworthy.wordpress.com there is more about Mary Beth's homeschool texts and a "Contact Us" page to send an email. On the website page for *Home Is a Feeling*, **you are invited** to view videos of Sally reading her original gift book along with other video clips of another Memory Care resident, Ms.Bonnie as she shares the book with a very special caretaker, Laura. **Please share your experience sharing *Home Is a Feeling* with your loved one (brief video clips welcome) using the Contact Me page of the website.**

www.ingramcontent.com/pod-product-compliance
Lightning Source LLC
Chambersburg PA
CBHW041608260326

41914CB00012B/1429